CKD STAGE 3 FOOD LIST

The Complete Beginner's Guide Ingredient list and Low sodium & Low Potassium Food to Avoid for People With Kidney Disease

Harley W. Norman

Copyright © 2024 by Harley W. Norman

All rights reserved

No part of this publication may be reproduced, stored in a retrieval system. or transmitted. in and form or by any means, electronic, mechanical, photocopying, recording, or otherwise, without the prior written permission of the author. The information in this eBook is true and complete to the best

of our knowledge. All recommendations are made without guarantee on the part of the author or publisher. The author and publisher disclaim any liability in connection with the use of this information.

Introduction

In the heart of a bustling city, there was a small, unassuming bookstore that held within its walls a treasure trove of knowledge, stories, and secrets. Among its prized possessions was a particular book that seemed to call out to those who needed it most. This book was titled, "The Lifesaver: Navigating CKD Stage 3 Through Your Plate."

The story begins with Alex, a vibrant individual in their early fifties, who had recently been diagnosed with Chronic Kidney Disease (CKD) Stage 3. The diagnosis came as a shock, leaving Alex feeling overwhelmed and unsure of how to manage their condition. The doctor had emphasized the importance of diet in slowing the progression of the disease, but the information given was dense, complex, and hard to follow.

One day, while wandering the aisles of the local bookstore, Alex stumbled upon the CKD Stage 3 food list book. The cover, showing a plate divided into colorful, kidney-friendly food sections, immediately caught their attention. Intrigued, Alex picked it up and began to flip through the pages.

The book was not just a food list; it was a comprehensive guide and a beacon of hope. It started with an empathetic introduction to CKD and its stages, particularly Stage 3, explaining the condition in a way that was both informative and comforting. It laid out the critical role of diet in managing CKD, setting the stage for the wealth of knowledge that followed.

What made the book truly stand out were the chapters on nutritional needs specific to CKD Stage 3, listing nutrients to limit and those to encourage, accompanied by a detailed food list that was both extensive and easy to navigate. Foods to avoid were clearly marked, taking away the guesswork and anxiety of meal planning.

Alex was particularly drawn to the sections on meal planning and preparation, which included sample meal plans and recipes tailored for CKD patients. The book made it clear that a kidney-friendly diet did not mean bland or boring meals. Instead, it opened up a world of flavors, ingredients, and cooking techniques designed to protect kidney function without sacrificing taste.

As Alex delved deeper, they found chapters on lifestyle considerations, managing the disease with diet, and even navigating dining out, ensuring that CKD Stage 3 patients could lead a full and active life. The appendices with a food diary template and a resource list for CKD patients were practical tools that promised to make the journey easier.

But what truly convinced Alex to buy the book was the realization that it was more than just a guide; it was a companion on a challenging journey. The book understood the fears, challenges, and questions that came with a CKD diagnosis and offered answers, guidance, and reassurance.

Purchasing "The Lifesaver: Navigating CKD Stage 3 Through Your Plate" was not just a transaction for Alex; it was a pivotal moment in their journey with CKD. It equipped them with the knowledge and confidence to manage their condition through diet, transforming fear into empowerment.

The story of Alex and the CKD Stage 3 food list book is a testament to the power of knowledge, the importance of tailored guidance, and the impact of understanding and managing one's health condition. It is a story that invites readers to discover how they too can navigate the challenges of CKD Stage 3, armed with the right information, support, and a plate full of hope.

Overview of Chronic Kidney Disease (CKD) and Its Stages

Chronic Kidney Disease (CKD) is a condition characterized by a gradual loss of kidney function over time. The kidneys, vital organs responsible for filtering wastes and excess fluids from the blood, which are then excreted through urine, become less effective in their role. This inefficiency can lead to the accumulation of harmful levels of fluid, electrolytes, and wastes in the body. CKD is measured in stages, from 1 to 5, based on the rate at which the kidneys filter blood, known as the glomerular filtration rate (GFR). Stage 3 CKD, a midpoint in the progression of kidney disease, is a critical phase where the kidneys are moderately damaged and have a reduced GFR of 30 to 59 ml/min. This stage is often where symptoms become more noticeable, and interventions, particularly dietary adjustments, become crucial in managing the disease's progression.

The dietary management of CKD, especially at Stage 3, focuses on reducing the kidneys' workload to slow the progression of damage. It involves a careful balance of nutrients to prevent further decline in kidney function while maintaining overall health. Key dietary adjustments include limiting intake of sodium, potassium, and phosphorus, which are harder for the kidneys to filter out at this stage. Protein intake also needs careful management; while excessive protein can burden the kidneys, it's essential to consume enough to maintain muscle mass and overall health.

A CKD Stage 3 food list typically includes fruits and vegetables with lower potassium levels, such as apples, berries, and carrots, while avoiding or limiting high-potassium foods like bananas, oranges, and potatoes. Whole grains, lean proteins, including fish and poultry, and low-phosphorus dairy alternatives are encouraged. Foods high in sodium and phosphorus, commonly found in processed and fast foods, should be avoided to help control blood pressure and prevent bone disease, a common complication of CKD.

Understanding the nutritional content of foods and reading labels becomes vital at this stage. The goal is to create a balanced plate that supports kidney health without depriving the body of necessary nutrients. Incorporating a variety of kidney-friendly foods not only aids in managing CKD but also contributes to a more enjoyable and sustainable diet.

Moreover, fluid intake may need to be monitored depending on the individual's fluid levels and kidney function. While staying hydrated is important, too much fluid can lead to complications in CKD Stage 3, such as hypertension and swelling.

Ultimately, managing CKD Stage 3 with a tailored food list and dietary plan is a proactive strategy to delay the progression to more advanced stages of kidney disease. It involves a holistic approach that considers the nutritional needs of the body while minimizing the strain on the kidneys. This dietary management, combined with regular monitoring of kidney function and consultations with healthcare professionals, plays a pivotal role in maintaining quality of life for individuals with CKD Stage 3.

Importance of Diet in Managing CKD Stage 3

Diet plays a crucial role in managing Chronic Kidney Disease (CKD) Stage 3, where the kidneys are moderately damaged and cannot filter blood as efficiently as they should. In this stage, making informed dietary choices is essential to slow the progression of the disease, minimize symptoms, and improve overall health outcomes. A CKD Stage 3 food list becomes an invaluable tool in this context, guiding patients towards foods that support kidney health while avoiding those that can exacerbate kidney damage.

One of the primary reasons diet is so important at this stage is its impact on the buildup of waste products and fluids in the body. As kidney function declines, the kidneys' ability to remove waste products from the blood decreases. This makes it critical to limit certain nutrients that can accumulate in the body and cause harm, such as sodium, potassium, and phosphorus. The CKD Stage 3 food list helps patients identify low-sodium foods to manage blood pressure and reduce swelling, as well as foods with appropriate levels of potassium and phosphorus to prevent heart issues and bone disease.

Protein intake is another key dietary consideration. While protein is an essential nutrient, excessive protein can increase the burden on the kidneys, leading to a faster decline in kidney function. The food list aids in selecting high-quality protein sources in quantities that meet, but do not exceed, the body's needs, balancing nutrition with kidney health.

Furthermore, the diet emphasizes the importance of consuming foods rich in antioxidants and anti-inflammatory compounds. Chronic kidney disease can be associated with increased levels of inflammation and oxidative stress, which contribute to the progression of kidney damage and other health issues like cardiovascular disease. Foods high in antioxidants, such as certain fruits and vegetables, can help reduce inflammation and protect the kidneys from further damage.

Fluid intake is also a consideration. While individuals with CKD Stage 3 may not need to restrict their fluid intake as much as those in later stages, it's important to monitor and adjust it based on the body's needs, especially in cases of swelling or heart disease. The food list can guide patients towards hydrating foods that also support kidney health.

In addition to managing these specific nutrients, the CKD Stage 3 food list supports overall nutritional health, ensuring patients receive a balanced diet that supports their overall health without overburdening the kidneys. It includes options for incorporating a variety of fruits, vegetables, whole grains, lean proteins, and healthy fats into the diet, which can help manage other health conditions commonly associated with CKD, such as diabetes and hypertension.

Ultimately, the CKD Stage 3 food list is more than just a list of foods to eat and avoid; it's a roadmap for navigating the dietary challenges of managing kidney disease. It empowers patients to make informed choices about their nutrition, leading to improved quality of life, delayed progression of CKD, and potentially avoiding the need for dialysis or a kidney transplant. By understanding and applying the principles behind the food list, patients can actively participate in their care and take control of their kidney health.

How to Use This Guide

Navigating through the complexities of Chronic Kidney Disease (CKD) Stage 3 requires careful consideration, especially when it comes to diet and nutrition. This guide is designed to empower individuals with CKD Stage 3 to make informed decisions about their dietary choices, ultimately helping to manage their condition and improve their quality of life. Understanding how to use this guide effectively is the first step towards taking control of your health and well-being.

Start by familiarizing yourself with the basics of CKD Stage 3, including the role that diet plays in managing this condition. The guide provides an overview of how certain foods impact kidney function, highlighting the importance of nutrients like sodium, potassium, phosphorus, and protein. It's crucial to grasp why some foods are encouraged and others are limited or avoided altogether. This foundational knowledge will help you understand the rationale behind the dietary recommendations that follow.

Dive into the food list section, which is the heart of this guide. It categorizes foods into safe options and those to limit or avoid. Use this section as a reference when planning meals, shopping for groceries, or eating out. The list is detailed and comprehensive, covering a wide range of food groups including vegetables, fruits, grains, proteins, dairy, and more. For each food item, there's information on its nutritional content and how it fits into a kidney-friendly diet.

Meal planning and preparation tips are invaluable components of the guide. These sections offer practical advice on how to incorporate the recommended foods into your daily meals. There's guidance on reading food labels, choosing the right cooking methods, and even suggestions for dining out without straying from your dietary goals. Use these tips to create varied and nutritious meals that cater to your personal preferences and lifestyle.

Recipes tailored to the dietary needs of CKD Stage 3 patients are a highlight. These recipes are designed to be both delicious and kidney-friendly, showing that a restrictive diet doesn't have to be boring or flavorless. Experiment with these recipes, adapting them as needed to suit your taste and nutritional requirements. Cooking your own meals gives you control over what you eat and is a positive step towards managing CKD.

Adjusting to dietary changes can be challenging, but the guide emphasizes the importance of patience and persistence. It suggests setting realistic goals, tracking your progress, and celebrating small victories. Remember, dietary management of CKD is a long-term commitment and a key aspect of your overall treatment plan.

Monitoring your health and kidney function is critical. The guide advises on how to work closely with your healthcare provider to track the progress of your condition and adjust your diet as necessary. Regular check-ups and tests will help determine if your dietary choices are effectively supporting your kidney health.

Finally, the guide is meant to be a living document that adapts to your evolving needs. Keep it accessible, revisit it frequently, and update it as your condition, lifestyle, and dietary recommendations change. Engage with support groups, healthcare professionals, and fellow CKD patients to share experiences and tips.

Using this guide to its fullest potential means actively engaging with its content, applying its recommendations to your daily life, and maintaining an open dialogue with your healthcare team. It's a tool that empowers you to make positive dietary choices, manage CKD Stage 3 more effectively, and lead a healthier, more vibrant life.

Understanding CKD Stage 3

Definition and Diagnosis

Chronic Kidney Disease (CKD) Stage 3 is a crucial juncture in the spectrum of kidney health, marking a moderate decline in kidney function. At this stage, the kidneys, vital organs responsible for filtering wastes and excess fluid from the blood, have suffered enough damage to affect their ability to perform efficiently, yet not so severe that the most drastic symptoms or need for renal replacement therapy, such as dialysis or transplantation, are present. The defining metric for diagnosing CKD Stage 3 is the glomerular filtration rate (GFR), a calculation based on serum creatinine levels, age, sex, and race, which estimates the rate of blood flow through the kidneys. A GFR of 30 to 59 ml/min per 1.73 m² is indicative of Stage 3 CKD, signaling a moderate reduction in kidney function.

The diagnosis of CKD Stage 3 often follows routine blood work that reveals elevated levels of creatinine or urea, indicating decreased kidney function. This stage may also be detected through proteinuria, the presence of excess protein in the urine, which is another marker of kidney damage. Many individuals at this stage begin to experience symptoms that can include fatigue, fluid retention, changes in urination patterns, and blood pressure fluctuations, though some may still remain asymptomatic.

Given the implications of CKD Stage 3 on health and lifestyle, including the need for dietary adjustments, the role of a comprehensive diagnostic process cannot be overstated. Upon suspicion or detection of CKD, further diagnostic tests such as urine tests for albumin (a type of protein) and imaging tests to visualize kidney structure may be employed to confirm the diagnosis and assess the extent of kidney damage.

Understanding the diagnosis of CKD Stage 3 is foundational to managing the disease, particularly through dietary interventions. The moderate reduction in kidney function necessitates a careful review of one's diet to manage the intake of certain nutrients and fluids that the kidneys can no longer handle efficiently. Adjustments typically involve limiting foods high in potassium, phosphorus, and sodium to avoid further stressing the kidneys. At the same time, protein consumption is moderated to reduce the buildup of waste products in the blood, while ensuring adequate intake to support overall health.

The focus on diet following a diagnosis of CKD Stage 3 underscores the importance of individualized dietary planning. Nutritional needs can vary widely among individuals based on factors such as residual kidney function, body size, and concurrent health conditions. Therefore, dietary recommendations often require the guidance of healthcare professionals, including dietitians specialized in renal nutrition, to ensure that the diet not only supports kidney health but also maintains nutritional balance.

In conclusion, the diagnosis of CKD Stage 3 marks a pivotal point where intervention through dietary management becomes a key component of care. It necessitates a nuanced understanding of the relationship between diet and kidney function, highlighting the need for individualized dietary guidance to slow the progression of kidney damage while supporting overall health and well-being.

Symptoms and Complications

Chronic Kidney Disease (CKD) Stage 3 is a critical juncture where the kidneys are moderately impaired, and the symptoms become more noticeable compared to the earlier stages. Individuals with CKD Stage 3 often experience fatigue, swelling in the hands and feet due to fluid retention, back pain located near the kidneys, and changes in urination patterns, such as foamy or dark urine. These symptoms arise because the kidneys can no longer efficiently filter waste and excess fluids from the body, leading to a build-up of toxins and imbalances in electrolytes.

As CKD progresses to Stage 3, complications can become more prominent and affect overall health. One significant complication is high blood pressure, which can further damage the kidneys and lead to cardiovascular diseases. Mineral and bone disorder, a condition in which there is an imbalance of calcium and phosphorus in the blood, can also occur, leading to bone pain and an increased risk of fractures. Anemia, characterized by a shortage of red blood cells, is another complication that can cause weakness and fatigue because the kidneys produce less erythropoietin, a hormone needed for red blood cell production.

Diet plays a crucial role in managing symptoms and preventing complications in CKD Stage 3. Adhering to a food list tailored for CKD can help control blood pressure, reduce fluid retention, and balance key nutrients, thereby alleviating some symptoms and reducing the risk of complications. For instance, limiting sodium intake is essential to manage blood pressure and reduce swelling. Avoiding high potassium foods can prevent hyperkalemia, a condition caused by too much potassium in the blood, which can affect heart function. Similarly, controlling phosphorus intake helps prevent mineral and bone disorders.

Moreover, a CKD Stage 3 food list emphasizes the importance of controlling protein intake. While protein is a vital nutrient, excessive amounts can increase the kidneys' workload, exacerbating kidney damage. However, it's important not to underconsume protein to avoid malnutrition. Finding the right balance is key, and high-quality proteins like fish, egg whites, and poultry are recommended because they produce fewer waste products during digestion.

Fluid intake also needs careful consideration in CKD Stage 3. While individuals may not need to restrict their fluid intake severely, it's essential to avoid excessive fluid intake to prevent fluid overload, which can lead to swelling and hypertension.

Incorporating kidney-friendly foods that are rich in antioxidants and anti-inflammatory properties can also support overall health and potentially slow the progression of CKD. These include berries, bell peppers, and garlic, which provide essential nutrients without overburdening the kidneys.

Managing symptoms and preventing complications in CKD Stage 3 involves a comprehensive approach that includes dietary modifications. Adhering to a CKD Stage 3 food list can help mitigate the symptoms of kidney disease, such as swelling and fatigue, and address complications like high blood pressure, mineral and bone disorder, and anemia. By carefully selecting foods and monitoring nutrient intake, individuals can support their kidney function and maintain their quality of life.

Monitoring and Managing CKD Stage 3

Chronic Kidney Disease (CKD) Stage 3 marks a critical juncture in the progression of kidney impairment, where the kidneys have moderately reduced function with a glomerular filtration rate (GFR) of 30 to 59 ml/min. At this stage, individuals may begin to notice symptoms such as fatigue, fluid retention, and changes in urination patterns, signaling the need for closer monitoring and proactive management to slow the disease's progression and mitigate symptoms. A cornerstone of managing CKD Stage 3 involves comprehensive monitoring of kidney function and adopting a tailored dietary approach to support kidney health.

Monitoring CKD Stage 3 entails regular consultations with healthcare professionals to assess kidney function through blood and urine tests. These tests measure levels of creatinine and urea, indicators of kidney health, and screen for proteinuria (excess protein in urine), a sign of kidney damage. Blood pressure monitoring is also essential, as hypertension can both contribute to and result from kidney disease. Achieving and maintaining target blood pressure levels can significantly reduce the risk of CKD progression.

Dietary management in CKD Stage 3 focuses on balancing nutrient intake to reduce the kidneys' workload and prevent further damage.

Sodium, potassium, phosphorus, and protein intake must be carefully managed. A diet low in sodium helps manage blood pressure, a critical aspect since hypertension can accelerate kidney damage. Limiting foods high in potassium and phosphorus is necessary to prevent complications associated with CKD, such as heart issues and bone disorders, as impaired kidneys can struggle to maintain the balance of these minerals.

Protein consumption requires a delicate balance; while excessive protein can increase the kidneys' filtering load, leading to further damage, it is vital for maintaining overall health. Guidance from a dietitian specialized in kidney disease can help individuals navigate the complexities of protein intake. This balance is crucial in CKD Stage 3, where dietary protein quality, not just quantity, becomes paramount.

A CKD Stage 3 food list is instrumental in guiding dietary choices. It typically includes fruits and vegetables with lower potassium content, grains, and cereals that are not enriched with added phosphorus, lean proteins, and dairy alternatives low in phosphorus and potassium. Reading food labels becomes an essential skill to identify added phosphorus, sodium, and potassium in packaged foods and avoid them.

Fluid intake in CKD Stage 3 also requires attention. While individuals with CKD Stage 3 do not usually need to limit their fluid intake unless they experience fluid retention or hypertension, staying adequately hydrated is crucial. However, it's essential to avoid excessive fluid intake, which can lead to swelling and increase blood pressure.

Education on CKD and nutritional counseling plays a significant role in managing CKD Stage 3. Understanding the impact of diet on kidney health and how to make informed food choices empowers individuals to take control of their health and can improve outcomes. Dietitians and healthcare providers can provide valuable resources, including detailed food lists, meal planning tips, and strategies for eating out, to help maintain a kidney-friendly diet.

Lifestyle modifications, including regular physical activity, smoking cessation, and weight management, complement dietary management in slowing CKD progression and improving quality of life. These changes can help reduce blood pressure, improve cardiovascular health, and support overall well-being.

Managing CKD Stage 3 effectively requires a multifaceted approach that includes regular monitoring of kidney function, tailored dietary management to reduce the kidneys' workload, and lifestyle modifications. By focusing on a balanced diet and closely monitoring their health, individuals with CKD Stage 3 can play a proactive role in managing their condition and potentially slowing its progression.

Nutritional Needs in CKD Stage 3

Overview of Nutritional Requirements

Managing Chronic Kidney Disease (CKD) Stage 3 through diet involves a nuanced understanding of nutritional requirements to slow the progression of kidney damage while maintaining overall health. The key is to balance nutrient intake to support kidney function without overloading the kidneys with substances they can no longer filter effectively. This delicate balance impacts how individuals with CKD Stage 3 should approach their daily food choices.

First and foremost, protein intake must be carefully managed. In the context of CKD, the body still requires protein for repair and maintenance, but excessive amounts can increase the kidneys' workload. High-quality proteins, such as those found in lean meats, fish, eggs, and plant-based sources like legumes, are recommended, but in controlled quantities. The aim is to meet the body's needs without exacerbating kidney stress.

Sodium intake requires strict monitoring to manage blood pressure, a crucial aspect of CKD management. High blood pressure can further damage kidney function, so limiting foods high in sodium, such as processed foods, canned soups, and salty snacks, is advised.

Seasonings and herbs can serve as alternatives to salt for flavoring dishes, helping to reduce sodium intake without sacrificing taste.

Potassium levels must also be regulated. While potassium is vital for nerve function and muscle control, damaged kidneys may struggle to maintain the right balance, potentially leading to dangerous heart rhythms. Foods high in potassium, such as bananas, oranges, potatoes, and tomatoes, should be consumed in moderation, and low-potassium alternatives like apples, berries, and zucchini are encouraged.

Phosphorus control is another cornerstone of dietary management in CKD Stage 3. Excess phosphorus can lead to bone and cardiovascular problems as damaged kidneys can't filter out phosphate efficiently. Foods high in phosphorus, including dairy products, nuts, seeds, and whole grains, should be limited. Phosphorus additives found in processed foods are particularly absorbable and should be avoided as much as possible.

Fluid intake may need adjustment based on individual needs and kidney function. While adequate hydration is important, too much fluid can lead to swelling, hypertension, and heart issues in CKD Stage 3 patients. Fluid needs can vary widely among individuals, so guidance from healthcare professionals is crucial.

Nutritional requirements in CKD Stage 3 also extend to vitamins and minerals. Some patients may need supplements due to dietary restrictions or altered kidney function affecting nutrient balance. However, vitamin and mineral supplementation should only be done under medical advice to avoid exacerbating kidney damage.

The dietary approach to managing CKD Stage 3 focuses on maintaining a balanced intake of these nutrients to support overall health without overburdening the kidneys. Adapting to these dietary changes can be challenging, but with the right guidance and a carefully curated food list, individuals can effectively manage their condition and maintain a good quality of life. Regular consultations with dietitians and healthcare providers are essential to tailor dietary plans to individual needs, monitor nutritional status, and adjust as necessary based on kidney function and overall health status.

Nutrients to Limit

For individuals navigating the complexities of Chronic Kidney Disease (CKD) Stage 3, understanding and managing dietary needs is pivotal. At this juncture of the disease, the kidneys are moderately impaired, necessitating adjustments in the consumption of certain nutrients to alleviate the kidneys' workload and slow the progression of CKD. The primary nutrients to monitor and limit include sodium, potassium, phosphorus, and proteins. These dietary adjustments are crucial in preventing the exacerbation of symptoms and complications associated with CKD.

Sodium is a mineral found abundantly in most diets, primarily through salt (sodium chloride). It plays a critical role in regulating blood pressure and fluid balance. However, in CKD Stage 3, the kidneys' diminished ability to filter and excrete sodium leads to its accumulation, causing fluid retention, hypertension, and swelling. This exacerbation of blood pressure can further damage kidney function. Patients are advised to limit their sodium intake to 2,000 milligrams per day or less, according to individual recommendations from healthcare providers. To achieve this, it is advisable to avoid high-sodium foods like processed meats, canned soups, and fast foods, and to opt for fresh, unprocessed foods while using herbs and spices for flavoring instead of salt.

Potassium is another mineral crucial for the proper function of nerve and muscle cells, including those in the heart. While potassium is necessary for health, too much potassium can be dangerous for people with CKD Stage 3 because their kidneys cannot excrete it effectively. High potassium levels in the blood can lead to hyperkalemia, a condition that can cause muscle weakness, fatigue, and heart problems. To manage potassium intake, it is important to limit high-potassium foods such as bananas, oranges, potatoes, spinach, and tomatoes. Instead, consuming lower-potassium alternatives like apples, berries, carrots, and green beans can help maintain balance.

Phosphorus, like potassium, is essential for bone health and energy production but becomes problematic when the kidneys fail to eliminate excess amounts from the blood. In CKD, high phosphorus levels can lead to bone and cardiovascular diseases by pulling calcium out of the bones, making them weak. Dietary phosphorus is found in foods like dairy products, nuts, seeds, beans, and whole grains. Limiting the intake of high-phosphorus foods and opting for alternatives such as rice milk, corn cereals, and non-whole grains can help manage phosphorus levels. Additionally, some patients may require phosphate binders, medications that bind to phosphorus in the gut so it can be eliminated from the body.

Proteins are the building blocks of the body, essential for growth, health, and repair. However, consuming more protein than the body needs can strain the kidneys because protein breakdown generates waste that must be filtered by the kidneys. In CKD Stage 3, moderating protein intake can reduce the kidneys' workload and help preserve kidney function. The recommended amount of protein varies based on the patient's health, activity level, and stage of CKD, necessitating individualized dietary planning with a healthcare provider or dietitian. High-quality proteins, which contain all the essential amino acids, are preferable. Sources include lean meats, fish, eggs, and plant-based options like quinoa and soy products.

Managing the intake of sodium, potassium, phosphorus, and proteins is integral to the dietary management of CKD Stage 3. A carefully curated CKD Stage 3 food list, developed in consultation with healthcare professionals, can guide patients in choosing foods that support their kidney health while ensuring their diet remains balanced and nutritious. This proactive approach to diet can significantly impact the quality of life for individuals with CKD Stage 3, helping to manage symptoms and delay the progression of kidney disease.

Nutrients to Encourage

In managing Chronic Kidney Disease (CKD) Stage 3, while certain dietary restrictions are crucial to reduce kidney strain, equally important is the focus on incorporating beneficial nutrients. These essential nutrients not only support overall health but also aid in managing CKD progression. Individuals with CKD Stage 3 should emphasize the intake of fiber, omega-3 fatty acids, and specific vitamins and minerals to optimize their kidney function and overall wellbeing.

Fiber plays a pivotal role in the dietary management of CKD Stage 3. Found in fruits, vegetables, whole grains, and legumes, fiber aids in digestion, helps regulate blood sugar levels, and can lower cholesterol, which are all beneficial for kidney health. For CKD patients, a fiber-rich diet also contributes to cardiovascular health and helps manage weight, reducing the risks associated with obesity and hypertension. Foods such as berries, carrots, and quinoa are excellent sources of fiber that are typically kidney-friendly and should be incorporated into a CKD Stage 3 food list.

Omega-3 Fatty Acids are crucial in reducing inflammation, a common issue in CKD which can contribute to the progression of kidney damage. Omega-3s also have a protective effect on the heart and blood vessels, reducing the risk of cardiovascular diseases, which CKD patients are particularly susceptible to. Fatty fish like salmon, mackerel, and sardines are excellent sources of omega-3 fatty acids. For those who prefer plant-based sources, flaxseeds, chia seeds, and walnuts can be valuable additions to the diet. Including these foods in a CKD Stage 3 diet can help mitigate inflammation and protect cardiovascular health.

When it comes to Vitamins and Minerals, it's essential for individuals with CKD Stage 3 to get a balance that supports kidney health without overburdening them. Certain vitamins and minerals need careful monitoring and management due to the kidneys' diminished ability to filter and maintain balance.

- Vitamin D is vital for bone health, especially in CKD, where imbalances of calcium and phosphorus can lead to bone disorders. However, vitamin D levels should be monitored and managed under medical supervision, as the kidneys play a role in activating vitamin D.
- Iron is another important mineral since CKD can often lead to anemia. Incorporating iron-rich foods like lean meats, beans, and spinach can help, though iron supplements should only be used under a healthcare provider's guidance.

- Calcium and Vitamin K are also essential for bone health. While calcium needs are individualized in CKD patients to avoid complications, vitamin K, found in green leafy vegetables, supports bone and cardiovascular health. It's important to balance the intake of these nutrients to avoid exacerbating any CKD-related complications.

It's crucial for individuals with CKD Stage 3 to consult with a dietitian or healthcare provider to tailor their intake of these nutrients according to their blood work and individual health needs. Monitoring levels of potassium and phosphorus, especially when increasing the intake of fruits, vegetables, and whole grains for their fiber content, is essential to prevent any adverse effects due to these nutrients' accumulation.

Managing nutritional needs in CKD Stage 3 involves a careful balance of encouraging certain nutrients while managing overall intake to ensure the kidneys are supported without being overwhelmed. Fiber, omega-3 fatty acids, and specific vitamins and minerals can have significant positive effects on the health of individuals with CKD Stage 3. Tailoring the diet to include these nutrients, under medical guidance, can help slow the progression of kidney disease and improve quality of life.

Fluid Intake

Managing fluid intake is a critical aspect of the nutritional needs for individuals with Chronic Kidney Disease (CKD) Stage 3. As the kidneys' ability to filter and remove excess fluids from the blood diminishes, careful monitoring of fluid consumption becomes necessary to prevent complications such as hypertension, swelling (edema), and heart strain. The relationship between fluid intake and diet in CKD Stage 3 is intricate, as many foods contain high levels of water and other fluids that must be accounted for in daily intake.

For those with CKD Stage 3, the general advice is to consume fluids according to thirst and monitor for signs of fluid overload or dehydration. Unlike earlier stages of CKD, where the kidneys might still manage fluid balance efficiently, Stage 3 often requires a more tailored approach to fluid consumption. This includes not only the direct intake of beverages but also recognizing the fluid content in fruits, vegetables, soups, and other moist foods.

The CKD Stage 3 food list plays a vital role in managing fluid intake. Foods with high water content, such as watermelon, cucumber, lettuce, and broth-based soups, can contribute significantly to overall fluid intake. While these foods are nutritious and can be part of a healthy kidney diet, their fluid content needs to be considered in the daily fluid allowance. Conversely, some foods and beverages might need to be limited due to their impact on fluid retention. For instance, foods high in sodium can increase thirst and promote fluid retention, complicating fluid management efforts.

Fluid intake recommendations can vary widely among individuals with CKD Stage 3, depending on their residual kidney function, presence of conditions like diabetes or heart disease, and the use of certain medications that affect fluid balance. Therefore, personalized advice from healthcare providers, including dietitians specializing in kidney health, is essential. They can offer guidance on how much fluid to consume daily, taking into account both beverages and the water content of foods.

Practical tips for managing fluid intake include measuring daily fluid consumption, using smaller cups or glasses, avoiding salty foods that increase thirst, and spreading fluid intake evenly throughout the day to avoid overburdening the kidneys at any one time. For individuals who experience thirst, sucking on ice chips, frozen grapes, or lemon slices can provide relief without significantly increasing fluid intake.

Monitoring for signs of fluid imbalance is also critical. Symptoms of fluid overload include sudden weight gain, swelling in the legs, ankles, or around the eyes, and high blood pressure. On the other hand, symptoms of dehydration, though less common in CKD Stage 3, include dry mouth, thirst, dark-colored urine, and dizziness.

Fluid intake management in CKD Stage 3 is a delicate balance that requires careful consideration of both beverages and the fluid content of foods. By adhering to a personalized fluid intake plan and making informed choices from the CKD Stage 3 food list, individuals can effectively manage their fluid balance, supporting overall health and slowing the progression of kidney disease. Collaboration with healthcare providers is key to tailoring fluid recommendations to each person's unique needs and circumstances, ensuring optimal care and quality of life.

Safe Foods for CKD Stage 3

Vegetables and Fruits

When managing Chronic Kidney Disease (CKD) Stage 3, diet plays a pivotal role in maintaining kidney health and preventing further decline in kidney function. Vegetables and fruits are essential components of a kidney-friendly diet due to their nutritional benefits, including being rich sources of vitamins, minerals, antioxidants, and fiber. However, it's important to choose varieties that align with the specific nutritional needs of CKD Stage 3, particularly regarding the limits on sodium, potassium, phosphorus, and proteins.

Below is a table that details safe vegetables and fruits for CKD Stage 3, including their benefits, nutritional information, and guidance on the mentioned nutrients.

Food	Benefits	Nutritional Information (per 100g)	Nutrient Limits
Apples	High in fiber and anti-inflammatory properties, good	Calories: 52, Potassium: 107 mg, Phosphorus:	Low in potassium, phosphorus,

Food	Benefits	Nutritional Information (per 100g)	Nutrient Limits
	for heart health.	11 mg, Sodium: 1 mg, Protein: 0.3g	sodium, and protein.
Berries	Rich in antioxidants, vitamins, and fiber. Good for cardiovascular health.	Calories: 43 (strawberries), Potassium: 153 mg, Phosphorus: 24 mg, Sodium: 1 mg, Protein: 0.7g (strawberries)	Generally low in potassium, phosphorus, and sodium. Protein varies by type.
Carrots	High in beta-carotene, fiber, and vitamins A, C, and K.	Calories: 41, Potassium: 320 mg, Phosphorus: 35 mg, Sodium: 69 mg, Protein: 0.9g	Moderate in potassium, low in phosphorus and sodium.
Cauliflower	A good source of vitamins C, K, and B6, and folate.	Calories: 25, Potassium: 299 mg, Phosphorus: 44 mg, Sodium: 30 mg, Protein: 1.9g	Moderate in potassium and phosphorus, low in sodium.

Food	Benefits	Nutritional Information (per 100g)	Nutrient Limits
Cabbage	Contains vitamin K, vitamin C, and fiber. Supports digestion and inflammation reduction.	Calories: 25, Potassium: 170 mg, Phosphorus: 26 mg, Sodium: 18 mg, Protein: 1.3g	Low in potassium, phosphorus, sodium, and protein.
Green beans	Rich in fiber, vitamins A, C, and K, and folate.	Calories: 31, Potassium: 209 mg, Phosphorus: 38 mg, Sodium: 6 mg, Protein: 1.8g	Moderate in potassium and phosphorus, low in sodium and protein.
Pineapple	Good source of vitamins C and B6, manganese, and antioxidants.	Calories: 50, Potassium: 109 mg, Phosphorus: 8 mg, Sodium: 1 mg, Protein: 0.5g	Low in potassium, phosphorus, sodium, and protein.
Grapes	High in vitamins C and K, antioxidants, and fiber.	Calories: 69, Potassium: 191 mg, Phosphorus: 20 mg, Sodium: 2	Low to moderate in potassium, low in phosphorus

Food	Benefits	Nutritional Information (per 100g)	Nutrient Limits
		mg, Protein: 0.7g	and sodium.

The table emphasizes foods with benefits suitable for CKD Stage 3 patients, such as anti-inflammatory properties and heart health support, without overloading the kidneys with excess nutrients they can no longer effectively filter. It's critical to manage portions and combine these foods with other kidney-friendly dietary elements to ensure a balanced intake of nutrients. Consulting with a healthcare provider or dietitian specializing in renal health is advised to tailor dietary choices to individual health needs and kidney function levels, allowing for adjustments in dietary plans as CKD progresses.

Grains and Cereals

In managing Chronic Kidney Disease (CKD) Stage 3, selecting the right grains and cereals is crucial as they form a significant part of a balanced diet. These foods provide essential energy, vitamins, minerals, and fiber, which can help manage CKD symptoms and potentially slow disease progression. However, it's important to choose grains and cereals that align with the dietary restrictions typical for CKD Stage 3, particularly concerning sodium, potassium, phosphorus, and protein levels.

The table below outlines safe and recommended grains and cereals for individuals with CKD Stage 3, highlighting their benefits and nutritional information to help adhere to nutrient limits.

Food Item	Benefits	Nutritional Information (per 1 cup serving)	Sodium (mg)	Potassium (mg)	Phosphorus (mg)	Protein (g)
White rice	Low in potassium and	Calories: 205, Carbs:	2	55	68	4.3

Food Item	Benefits	Nutritional Information (per 1 cup serving)	Sodium (mg)	Potassium (mg)	Phosphorus (mg)	Protein (g)
White bread	Lower in potassium and phosphorus, easy to digest than whole wheat	Calories: 79, Carbs: 15g, Fiber: 0.8g	150	28	20	2.2
Corn flakes	Fortified with vitamins, low in phosphorus	Calories: 100, Carbs: 24g, Fiber: 1g	200	45	20	2
Buckwh	High in	Calories:	3.5	148	118	5.7

Food Item	Benefits	Nutritional Information (per 1 cup serving)	Sodium (mg)	Potassium (mg)	Phosphorus (mg)	Protein (g)
eat	protein for a grain, good source of energy	155, Carbs: 33g, Fiber: 4.5g				
Pasta (refined)	Energy-rich, low in potassium and phosphorus	Calories: 220, Carbs: 43g, Fiber: 2.5g	1	63	72	8
Oatmeal	Good source of energy and fiber, low in	Calories: 158, Carbs: 27g, Fiber: 4g	115	163	180	6

Food Item	Benefits	Nutritional Information (per 1 cup serving)	Sodium (mg)	Potassium (mg)	Phosphorus (mg)	Protein (g)
Cream of Wheat	Provides iron and calcium, low in sodium and potassium	Calories: 126, Carbs: 27g, Fiber: 1.3g	83	95	176	3.6

Key Considerations for CKD Stage 3:

- **Sodium:** Managing sodium intake is crucial for CKD patients to avoid hypertension and fluid retention. It's advisable to choose grains and cereals that are low in sodium or sodium-free. Cooking grains from their unprocessed forms can help control sodium content, as pre-packaged products often contain added sodium.
- **Potassium:** While potassium is an essential mineral, CKD Stage 3 patients may need to limit its intake to avoid hyperkalemia, which can lead to heart complications. White rice and refined pasta are lower potassium options.

- **Phosphorus:** Phosphorus management is vital in CKD to prevent bone disease and cardiovascular issues. Choosing grains with lower phosphorus levels and avoiding or limiting whole grains can be beneficial.
- **Protein:** Protein needs in CKD Stage 3 should be carefully managed. Adequate protein is essential for health, but excessive intake can increase the kidneys' workload. Buckwheat and pasta provide moderate amounts of protein suitable for a CKD diet.

Selecting the right grains and cereals is an essential part of managing CKD Stage 3, aiding in dietary adherence and contributing to overall health without overburdening the kidneys. By focusing on grains and cereals that fit within the recommended nutritional limits for sodium, potassium, phosphorus, and protein, individuals with CKD Stage 3 can enjoy a varied diet that supports kidney health and well-being. Always consult with a healthcare provider or dietitian to tailor dietary choices to individual health needs and dietary restrictions.

Protein Sources

Managing protein intake is crucial for individuals with Chronic Kidney Disease (CKD) Stage 3, as it can help slow the progression of kidney damage while ensuring the body receives the nutrients it needs for overall health. The dietary approach in CKD Stage 3 involves selecting high-quality protein sources that are lower in sodium, potassium, phosphorus, and moderate in protein content to prevent overloading the kidneys.

Here's a detailed table outlining safe protein sources for CKD Stage 3, including their benefits, nutritional information, and nutrient limits.

Protein Source	Benefits	Nutritional Information (per 100g serving)	Sodium (mg)	Potassium (mg)	Phosphorus (mg)	Protein (g)
Egg Whites	High-quality protein with low	Calories: 52, Fat: 0.2g, Carbs: 0.7g	166	163	5	11

Protein Source	Benefits	Nutritional Information (per 100g serving)	Sodium (mg)	Potassium (mg)	Phosphorus (mg)	Protein (g)
	phosphorus, making it kidney-friendly.					
Chicken Breast	Lean protein source, low in phosphorus and potassium.	Calories: 165, Fat: 3.6g, Carbs: 0g	74	256	195	31
Fish (e.g., Cod)	Rich in omega-3 fatty acids, beneficial for heart	Calories: 105, Fat: 0.9g, Carbs: 0g	54	244	203	23

Protein Source	Benefits	Nutritional Information (per 100g serving)	Sodium (mg)	Potassium (mg)	Phosphorus (mg)	Protein (g)
Cottage Cheese (Low-sodium)	health. Low in phosphorus. Good source of calcium and protein. Choose low-sodium versions to minimize kidney strain.	Calories: 98, Fat: 4.3g, Carbs: 3.4g	15	104	159	11

Protein Source	Benefits	Nutritional Information (per 100g serving)	Sodium (mg)	Potassium (mg)	Phosphorus (mg)	Protein (g)
Tofu (Soft)	Plant-based protein, low in potassium and sodium, suitable for a kidney-friendly diet.	Calories: 61, Fat: 3.7g, Carbs: 2.3g	7	121	120	7

Key Points:

- **Egg Whites**: Ideal for those who need to control phosphorus intake closely, egg whites offer a high-quality protein source without the added burden of phosphorus found in the yolks.

- **Chicken Breast**: As a staple lean meat, skinless chicken breast is an excellent choice for a low-phosphorus and low-potassium diet, essential for CKD management.
- **Fish (e.g., Cod)**: Not only is fish a great protein source, but it also provides omega-3 fatty acids, which are important for cardiovascular health, a consideration for CKD patients.
- **Cottage Cheese (Low-sodium)**: Dairy can be high in phosphorus, but low-sodium cottage cheese offers a way to enjoy dairy protein with less risk. It's important to monitor portion sizes to keep phosphorus levels in check.
- **Tofu (Soft)**: For those on a plant-based diet or looking to reduce animal protein intake, tofu is an excellent low-potassium and low-sodium option that can be incorporated into various dishes.

Considerations:

When managing CKD Stage 3 through diet, it's essential to consider not just the individual nutrient limits but also the overall dietary pattern. Monitoring serving sizes is crucial, as consuming large quantities of even low-phosphorus or low-potassium foods can lead to nutrient accumulation. Working closely with a dietitian can help tailor a meal plan that balances protein needs with the limitations required to protect kidney function. This approach ensures that dietary management of CKD Stage 3 not only supports kidney health but also maintains overall nutritional balance.

Dairy and Dairy Alternatives

For individuals with Chronic Kidney Disease (CKD) Stage 3, dietary management is crucial to slowing disease progression and maintaining overall health. Dairy products and their alternatives play a significant role in this dietary management due to their nutritional content. However, considering the need to limit certain nutrients like sodium, potassium, phosphorus, and protein, choices within this category must be made carefully.

Below is a detailed table outlining various dairy and dairy alternative options, including their benefits, nutritional information, and how they align with the nutrient limits important for individuals with CKD Stage 3.

Food Item	Benefit	Nutritional Information (per 100g)	Nutrient Limit Considerations
Low-Fat Milk	Provides calcium, vitamin D, and protein. Essential for bone health	Calcium: 125 mg, Phosphorus: 95 mg, Potassium: 150 mg,	Lower in phosphorus and protein than whole milk, making it a better option for CKD Stage 3. Still,

Food Item	Benefit	Nutritional Information (per 100g)	Nutrient Limit Considerations
	and muscle function.	Sodium: 50 mg, Protein: 3.4 g	intake should be moderated due to phosphorus.
Rice Milk (Unenriched)	A low phosphorus and potassium alternative to dairy milk. Offers a good option for those needing to limit these minerals.	Calcium: 28 mg, Phosphorus: 29 mg, Potassium: 69 mg, Sodium: 39 mg, Protein: 0.3 g	Very low in protein and phosphorus, suitable for CKD Stage 3 diets. However, some brands may add minerals, so label reading is essential.
Almond Milk (Unsweetened)	Low in calories and free of saturated fats. Contains added calcium	Calcium: 450 mg, Phosphorus: 20 mg, Potassium: 120 mg,	Excellent for limiting phosphorus and protein. Keep an eye on added minerals and choose unsweetened

Food Item	Benefit	Nutritional Information (per 100g)	Nutrient Considerations
Greek Yogurt (Non-fat)	High in protein, which can help maintain muscle mass. Also provides probiotics for gut health.	and vitamin D. Sodium: 150 mg, Protein: 1 g Calcium: 110 mg, Phosphorus: 141 mg, Potassium: 141 mg, Sodium: 36 mg, Protein: 10 g	versions to avoid extra sugar. Higher in protein; thus, portion control is vital. Opt for non-fat to reduce phosphorus intake.
Cottage Cheese (Low-sodium)	Source of protein and calcium. Versatile in use, from snacks to main dishes.	Calcium: 83 mg, Phosphorus: 159 mg, Potassium: 104 mg, Sodium: 406 mg, Protein: 11 g	Choose low-sodium versions to manage sodium intake. High in protein, so monitor portion sizes.

Food Item	Benefit	Nutritional Information (per 100g)	Nutrient Limit Considerations
Soy Milk	Offers a plant-based protein source, along with vitamins and minerals. Particularly high in calcium if fortified.	Calcium: 300 mg, Phosphorus: 50 mg, Potassium: 118 mg, Sodium: 49 mg, Protein: 3.3 g	A good alternative for those limiting dairy. Check for unenriched versions to avoid excess phosphorus.
Hard Cheeses (Cheddar)	Rich in calcium and protein. Can add flavor to dishes in small amounts.	Calcium: 721 mg, Phosphorus: 512 mg, Potassium: 98 mg, Sodium: 621 mg, Protein: 25 g	High in sodium and phosphorus, which necessitates very limited consumption. Opt for small amounts as a flavor enhancer rather than a main component of meals.

Key Considerations:

- **Phosphorus:** Dairy products are a significant source of phosphorus, which needs to be limited in CKD Stage 3 to prevent bone disease and maintain kidney function.
- **Potassium:** While necessary for nerve function and muscle control, excessive potassium can be harmful if kidney function is compromised.
- **Sodium:** High sodium intake can raise blood pressure, leading to further kidney damage and cardiovascular issues.
- **Protein:** Protein needs are individualized in CKD. While essential for maintaining muscle mass and overall health, too much can increase kidney burden.

When incorporating dairy and dairy alternatives into a CKD Stage 3 diet, it's crucial to balance nutritional benefits with the need to limit certain nutrients. Selections should be made based on individual nutritional needs, preferences, and guidance from healthcare professionals, including dietitians specializing

Fats and Oils

In managing Chronic Kidney Disease (CKD) Stage 3 through diet, the types of fats and oils consumed play a significant role in overall health and kidney function. Choosing the right fats and limiting certain nutrients, including sodium, potassium, phosphorus, and proteins, are key considerations.

Here's a detailed look at fats and oils beneficial for CKD Stage 3, incorporating their health benefits, nutritional information, and how they align with nutrient limitations.

Fat/Oil Type	Health Benefits	Nutritional Information (per 1 tablespoon unless otherwise noted)	Sodium (mg)	Potassium (mg)	Phosphorus (mg)	Protein (g)
Olive Oil	Rich in monounsaturated fats; improves heart health	Calories: 119 Fat: 13.5g (Saturated: 1.9g, Monounsatur	0.3	0.1	0	0

Fat/Oil Type	Health Benefits	Nutritional Information (per 1 tablespoon unless otherwise noted)	Sodium (mg)	Potassium (mg)	Phosphorus (mg)	Protein (g)
	by lowering bad cholesterol levels. Contains antioxidants.	ated: 9.9g, Polyunsaturated: 1.4g)				
Canola Oil	High in omega-3 and omega-6 fatty acids; promotes heart health and has anti-inflammatory properties.	Calories: 124 Fat: 14g (Saturated: 1g, Monounsaturated: 8.9g, Polyunsaturated: 3.9g)	0	0	0	0
Flaxseed Oil	High in alpha-	Calories: 120 Fat: 13.6g	0	0	0	0

Fat/Oil Type	Health Benefits	Nutritional Information (per 1 tablespoon unless otherwise noted)	Sodium (mg)	Potassium (mg)	Phosphorus (mg)	Protein (g)
	linolenic acid, a type of omega-3 fatty acid; supports heart health and may help reduce inflammation.	(Saturated: 1.2g, Monounsaturated: 2.5g, Polyunsaturated: 9.2g)				
Walnut Oil	Rich in polyunsaturated fats and omega-3 fatty acids; good for heart health	Calories: 120 Fat: 13.6g (Saturated: 1.3g, Monounsaturated: 2.8g, Polyunsaturated	0	0	0	0

Fat/Oil Type	Health Benefits	Nutritional Information (per 1 tablespoon unless otherwise noted)	Sodium (mg)	Potassium (mg)	Phosphorus (mg)	Protein (g)
Avocado Oil	High in monounsaturated fats; lowers cholesterol, improves heart health, and has high smoke point for cooking.	Calories: 124 Fat: 14g (Saturated: 1.6g, Monounsaturated: 9.9g, Polyunsaturated: 1.9g) and may improve blood sugar levels. ed: 8.9g)	0	0	0	0

Key Points:

- **Health Benefits**: The fats and oils listed are predominantly rich in monounsaturated and polyunsaturated fats, including omega-3 and omega-6 fatty acids. These fats are essential for maintaining heart health, reducing inflammation, and managing cholesterol levels, all of which are crucial for individuals with CKD Stage 3.
- **Nutritional Information**: Each of these oils contains little to no sodium, potassium, phosphorus, and protein, making them suitable for a CKD diet. They provide healthy fats without contributing to the nutrient limitations typically necessary for CKD management.
- **Sodium, Potassium, Phosphorus, and Protein Limits**: For CKD patients, managing intake of these nutrients is critical to prevent further kidney damage and other complications. The oils listed contribute negligibly to these nutrients, making them a safe choice for inclusion in a CKD Stage 3 diet.

When incorporating these fats and oils into a CKD Stage 3 diet, it's important to use them in moderation due to their high calorie content. They can be used in cooking, salad dressings, and food preparation to enhance flavor and nutritional value without compromising kidney health. Additionally, replacing saturated fats found in butter, lard, and fatty meats with these healthier fats can further protect against cardiovascular disease and support overall well-being in individuals with CKD Stage 3.

Beverages

In the management of Chronic Kidney Disease (CKD) Stage 3, careful selection of beverages is crucial. Beverages can significantly affect the body's balance of key nutrients and fluids, necessitating careful consideration to avoid exacerbating kidney damage.

This table provides a comprehensive guide on safe beverage choices, including their benefits, nutritional content, and their alignment with the nutrient limits recommended for individuals with CKD Stage 3, focusing on sodium, potassium, phosphorus, and protein levels.

Beverage Type	Benefits	Nutritional Information (per 8 oz unless specified)	Nutrient Limits: Sodium, Potassium, Phosphorus, Protein
Water	Hydrates without adding sodium, potassium, or phosphorus.	0 mg Sodium, 0 mg Potassium, 0 mg Phosphorus, 0 g Protein	Ideal for managing fluid intake without affecting electrolyte balance.

Beverage Type	Benefits	Nutritional Information (per 8 oz unless specified)	Nutrient Limits: Sodium, Potassium, Phosphorus, Protein
Cranberry Juice (Low Sugar)	May help prevent urinary tract infections; antioxidant properties.	5 mg Sodium, 200 mg Potassium, 0 mg Phosphorus, 0 g Protein	Low in sodium and phosphorus; watch for potassium in portion control.
Apple Juice	Provides hydration with a lower potassium content than other fruit juices.	10 mg Sodium, 150 mg Potassium, 20 mg Phosphorus, 0 g Protein	Lower potassium option for a fruit juice.
Lemonade (Homemade with no added sugar)	Offers vitamin C; can be made with little to no sodium.	5 mg Sodium, 50 mg Potassium, 0 mg Phosphorus, 0 g Protein	A refreshing choice with minimal potassium and no phosphorus.

Beverage Type	Benefits	Nutritional Information (per 8 oz unless specified)	Nutrient Limits: Sodium, Potassium, Phosphorus, Protein
Brewed Coffee (Black, without additives)	Contains antioxidants; may reduce risk of certain diseases.	5 mg Sodium, 116 mg Potassium, 0 mg Phosphorus, 0.3 g Protein	Moderate potassium; limit quantity to control potassium intake.
Tea (Black or Green, unsweetened)	Antioxidant properties; may improve heart health.	5 mg Sodium, 88 mg Potassium, 0 mg Phosphorus, 0 g Protein	Lower in potassium than coffee; choose green for even lower potassium levels.
Sparkling Water (Unflavored, no additives)	Provides a sensation of soda without sodium,	0 mg Sodium, 0 mg Potassium, 0 mg Phosphorus, 0	Safe for maintaining fluid balance, offering a soda-like

Beverage Type	Benefits	Nutritional Information (per 8 oz unless specified)	Nutrient Limits: Sodium, Potassium, Phosphorus, Protein
	potassium, phosphorus.	or g Protein	experience without the risk.

Note: Nutritional values are approximate and can vary by brand and preparation. It's important to read labels for the most accurate information.

This table emphasizes beverages that are generally safe for individuals managing CKD Stage 3, highlighting the importance of selecting drinks that minimize the intake of sodium, potassium, phosphorus, and protein to prevent further kidney damage. By choosing beverages wisely, patients can enjoy varied and enjoyable options while adhering to dietary guidelines designed to support kidney health. It's crucial, however, to consult with healthcare providers or dietitians to personalize beverage choices based on individual health status, nutritional needs, and kidney function.

Foods to Avoid or Limit

High Sodium Foods

For individuals managing Chronic Kidney Disease (CKD) Stage 3, monitoring and limiting sodium intake is crucial. Sodium, a mineral found in many foods, is essential for bodily functions but in excess can lead to high blood pressure, swelling (edema), and further strain on the kidneys, exacerbating CKD progression. The kidneys play a pivotal role in maintaining sodium balance, but when their function is compromised, as in CKD Stage 3, the body's ability to regulate sodium and fluid levels diminishes. Consequently, a diet low in sodium is recommended to help manage blood pressure and reduce the risk of kidney damage progression.

Below is a table outlining high sodium foods that individuals with CKD Stage 3 should avoid or limit, including reasons for avoidance and examples of such foods:

Food Category	Reason to Avoid	Examples
Processed	High in sodium and	Bacon, sausages, deli

Food Category	Reason to Avoid	Examples
Meats	preservatives, contributing to increased blood pressure and fluid retention, which can overburden weakened kidneys.	meats, hot dogs
Canned Soups	Often contain large amounts of sodium as a preservative, which can exacerbate hypertension and kidney strain.	Cream of mushroom, chicken noodle, minestrone, beef broth
Fast Foods	Generally high in sodium and unhealthy fats, contributing to poor heart health and complicating fluid balance.	Burgers, fries, chicken nuggets, taco salads
Snack Foods	Typically loaded with sodium to enhance flavor and shelf life, increasing risk of high blood pressure and edema.	Potato chips, pretzels, crackers, salted nuts
Frozen Dinners	Contain high levels of sodium to preserve taste and extend shelf life, posing risks to	Frozen pizza, microwaveable entrees, frozen burritos

Food Category	Reason to Avoid	Examples
	blood pressure control and kidney health.	
Condiments & Sauces	Even small amounts can significantly increase the sodium content of meals, potentially leading to hypertension and fluid retention.	Soy sauce, ketchup, barbecue sauce, salad dressings
Pickled Foods	The pickling process involves large amounts of sodium, contributing to increased sodium intake which can aggravate blood pressure and fluid balance issues.	Pickles, olives, pickled vegetables
Salted and Seasoned	The use of seasoning blends and table salt adds considerable sodium to dishes, which can exacerbate health issues related to CKD Stage 3.	Table salt, garlic salt, taco seasoning, seasoning packets for pasta, rice, and noodle dishes

For individuals with CKD Stage 3, focusing on fresh, whole foods and using herbs and spices for flavoring instead of salt can significantly reduce sodium intake, helping to manage blood pressure and reduce the risk of further kidney damage. Consulting with a healthcare provider or dietitian can provide personalized guidance on dietary modifications that support kidney health, including strategies for reducing sodium consumption.

High Potassium Foods

In managing Chronic Kidney Disease (CKD) Stage 3, particular attention must be given to dietary potassium levels. This is because the kidneys play a critical role in maintaining the body's potassium balance, and when their function is impaired, potassium can accumulate in the blood, leading to hyperkalemia. Hyperkalemia is a serious condition that can affect heart rhythm and increase the risk of heart problems.

Therefore, individuals with CKD Stage 3 are often advised to limit their intake of high-potassium foods. The following table outlines foods that are high in potassium and suggests why they should be avoided or limited, along with examples of these foods.

Food Category	Why to Avoid or Limit	Examples of High-Potassium Foods
Fruits	Fruits are natural sources of potassium, which can contribute to elevated levels of potassium in the blood, potentially leading to hyperkalemia.	Bananas, oranges, apricots, dates, raisins, prunes, avocado, and melons (such as cantaloupe and honeydew).

Food Category	Why to Avoid or Limit	Examples of High-Potassium Foods
Vegetables	Similar to fruits, many vegetables are potassium-rich. Consuming large quantities can increase potassium intake significantly.	Potatoes (and sweet potatoes), tomatoes (and tomato-based products, such as sauces and juices), spinach, and beet greens.
Legumes	Legumes are nutritious but also high in potassium, making them a concern for individuals monitoring their potassium levels.	Kidney beans, black beans, lentils, and chickpeas.
Nuts and Seeds	Nuts and seeds are healthy snack options but are high in potassium, which can be problematic for those with reduced kidney function.	Almonds, pistachios, sunflower seeds, and pumpkin seeds.
Dairy Products	Dairy products are good calcium sources but also contain significant potassium amounts, which	Milk, yogurt, and cheese.

Food Category	Why to Avoid or Limit	Examples of High-Potassium Foods
	need to be limited in a kidney-friendly diet.	
Whole Grains	Whole grains are recommended for their fiber content, but some types are also high in potassium, requiring moderation in intake.	Bran cereals, whole wheat bread, and brown rice.
Meat and Fish	While necessary for protein, certain meats and fish are higher in potassium and should be consumed in moderation.	Beef, pork, salmon, and cod.
Beverages	Some beverages can have high potassium levels and contribute to overall potassium intake, necessitating careful selection.	Coconut water, orange juice, and certain sports drinks.

For individuals with CKD Stage 3, it is crucial to balance nutrition with the need to avoid excessive potassium intake. Dietitians often recommend substituting high-potassium foods with lower-potassium alternatives to maintain a healthy and balanced diet without compromising kidney health. For example, instead of bananas or oranges, one might opt for apples or berries. Similarly, cauliflower or carrots can replace high-potassium vegetables like potatoes or tomatoes.

Monitoring and adjusting dietary potassium is a key component of managing CKD Stage 3, aimed at preventing complications associated with hyperkalemia. Regular consultations with healthcare providers and dietitians can help individuals tailor their diet to their specific needs, ensuring they receive adequate nutrition while keeping potassium levels in check.

High Phosphorus Foods

Managing phosphorus intake is crucial for individuals with Chronic Kidney Disease (CKD) Stage 3, as the kidneys' ability to filter excess phosphorus begins to decline. High phosphorus levels in the blood can lead to bone and cardiovascular issues, making it important to avoid or limit certain foods rich in this mineral. The following table outlines high phosphorus foods that individuals with CKD Stage 3 should avoid or limit, including reasons for avoidance and examples of such foods:

Food Category	Reason to Avoid or Limit	Examples
Dairy Products	Dairy products are high in phosphorus, which can be hard for weakened kidneys to filter out, leading to an increased risk of bone disease and calcium buildup in blood vessels.	Milk, cheese, yogurt, ice cream
Processed Foods and Colas	These contain phosphorous additives that are almost completely absorbed by the body, potentially leading to elevated	Fast foods, ready-to-eat meals, cola soft drinks

Food Category	Reason to Avoid or Limit	Examples
	phosphorus levels.	
Nuts and Seeds	Although they are considered healthy, nuts and seeds are high in phosphorus, which can contribute to phosphorus build-up in the body when kidney function is compromised.	Almonds, peanuts, sunflower seeds, pumpkin seeds
Meats and Poultry	Certain meats and poultry are high in natural phosphorus. Furthermore, processed and enhanced meats can have added phosphates, making them even more problematic.	Organ meats, processed meats (e.g., sausages, deli meats)
Seafood	Seafood is naturally high in phosphorus, and just like with meats, some processed seafood can contain added phosphates.	Salmon, sardines, scallops, shrimp
Legumes	Beans, lentils, and other legumes are nutrient-dense foods but also	Beans (black, kidney),

Food Category	Reason to Avoid or Limit	Examples
	contain high amounts of phosphorus, necessitating moderation in consumption.	chickpeas, lentils
Whole Grains	Whole grains are preferred over refined grains for their nutrient content, but they also have higher phosphorus levels, requiring attention to portion sizes.	Whole wheat bread, bran cereals, oatmeal
Certain Vegetables	While most vegetables are kidney-friendly, some have higher phosphorus content and should be consumed in moderation.	Potatoes (if not leached), sweet potatoes, tomatoes

For individuals with CKD Stage 3, it's important to work with a healthcare provider or dietitian to develop a personalized diet plan. This plan should consider the individual's overall health, kidney function, and nutritional needs to manage phosphorus intake effectively while ensuring a balanced diet. Adjustments in dietary phosphorus are essential not just for kidney health but for the prevention of complications associated with elevated phosphorus levels, such as heart problems and bone disease.

Foods High in Saturated and Trans Fats

In managing Chronic Kidney Disease (CKD) Stage 3, diet plays a crucial role in slowing the disease's progression and minimizing complications. Among dietary considerations, limiting the intake of foods high in saturated and trans fats is essential. These fats can exacerbate cardiovascular issues, a common concern in individuals with CKD, by contributing to the buildup of plaque in the arteries and increasing the risk of heart disease. Moreover, diets high in unhealthy fats can lead to weight gain and increased blood pressure, further burdening the kidneys.

Below is a table outlining examples of foods high in saturated and trans fats, reasons to avoid them in the context of CKD Stage 3, and healthier alternatives.

Food Category	Examples to Avoid	Why to Avoid	Healthier Alternatives
Meats	Fatty cuts of beef, pork, and lamb; bacon; sausages	Saturated fats in these meats can increase LDL (bad) cholesterol, posing a risk to heart health. Excess protein	Lean meats, such as chicken breast or turkey; plant-based proteins like lentils and

Food Category	Examples to Avoid	Why to Avoid	Healthier Alternatives
		intake can also stress the kidneys.	beans.
Dairy Products	Butter; cream; full-fat cheese; regular ice cream	High in saturated fat, contributing to cholesterol levels and cardiovascular risk. Also, dairy products can be high in phosphorus.	Low-fat or non-fat dairy alternatives; almond, soy, or rice milk.
Snack Foods	Chips; cookies; pastries; commercially baked goods	Often contain trans fats (partially hydrogenated oils), which can raise LDL cholesterol and lower HDL (good) cholesterol, worsening heart health.	Fruits; nuts; homemade snacks with healthy fats, like avocado.

Food Category	Examples to Avoid	Why to Avoid	Healthier Alternatives
Fast Foods	Fried chicken; French fries; burgers; pizza	High in both saturated and trans fats, contributing to unhealthy weight gain, increased blood pressure, and higher risk of heart disease.	Grilled items; salads with lean protein; whole grain options.
Cooking Fats	Margarine sticks; lard; palm oil	Contain high levels of saturated and/or trans fats, impacting cardiovascular health negatively.	Olive oil; canola oil; other vegetable oils high in unsaturated fats.

For individuals with CKD Stage 3, it is not just about avoiding certain foods but making informed dietary choices that support kidney health and overall well-being. Substituting unhealthy fats with healthier options can significantly impact managing CKD and preventing its progression to more advanced stages. Incorporating a variety of nutrient-dense, kidney-friendly foods into the diet can help maintain optimal health while navigating the complexities of CKD Stage 3.

Meal Planning and Preparation

Reading Food Labels

Reading food labels is a crucial skill for anyone managing Chronic Kidney Disease (CKD) Stage 3, as it enables individuals to make informed choices about the foods they consume. This task becomes particularly important given the dietary restrictions associated with CKD, such as limiting sodium, potassium, phosphorus, and certain proteins. Understanding how to interpret the information presented on food labels can help maintain a balanced diet while preventing further kidney damage.

When examining a food label, the first section to consider is the serving size, which indicates the amount of food the nutritional information pertains to. This is essential for understanding the quantity of nutrients in a typical portion and ensuring that intake aligns with dietary recommendations for CKD management. For individuals with CKD Stage 3, keeping track of serving sizes helps manage nutrient intake more accurately, especially for those nutrients that need to be limited.

Next, the focus should shift to the nutritional facts panel, which lists the amount of various nutrients. Sodium is one of the primary concerns for CKD patients due to its role in elevating blood pressure, a common complication of kidney disease. Foods low in sodium, generally defined as containing less than 140 mg per serving, are preferable. Since the kidneys' ability to filter potassium and phosphorus is compromised in CKD Stage 3, it is also important to monitor the intake of these minerals. However, not all food labels list potassium and phosphorus, so it may be necessary to research or consult additional resources to determine their levels in certain foods.

Protein content is another critical component of the label. While protein is a necessary part of the diet, excessive intake can burden the kidneys. Therefore, selecting foods with appropriate protein levels, in consultation with a healthcare provider or dietitian, is key to managing CKD Stage 3 effectively.

In addition to these specific nutrients, the overall calorie content and the types of fats in foods are also important. Choosing foods with healthier fats, such as monounsaturated and polyunsaturated fats, over those high in saturated and trans fats can help manage cholesterol levels and reduce the risk of heart disease, another concern for individuals with CKD.

Finally, the ingredients list on the food label provides insight into the food's composition, including additives that may be best avoided, such as sodium phosphates. The ingredients are listed in order of quantity, from highest to lowest, offering an additional layer of information to assess the suitability of a food item for a kidney-friendly diet.

Incorporating the practice of reading food labels into meal planning and preparation is a proactive step in managing CKD Stage 3. It not only assists in adhering to dietary restrictions but also empowers individuals to make choices that support their kidney health and overall well-being. By understanding and utilizing the information on food labels, people with CKD can maintain a diet that is both nutritious and aligned with their health needs, contributing to the management of their condition and the prevention of its progression.

Cooking and Preparing Meals at Home

Cooking and preparing meals at home for those managing Chronic Kidney Disease (CKD) Stage 3 requires careful planning and a thoughtful approach to ingredients and cooking methods. A CKD Stage 3 food list serves as a guide to selecting kidney-friendly foods that support health while minimizing the burden on the kidneys. This approach helps in tailoring meals to the nutritional needs specific to CKD, focusing on controlling the intake of sodium, potassium, phosphorus, and protein, and managing fluid levels.

When planning meals, the emphasis is on fresh, whole foods and avoiding processed items that often contain high levels of sodium, phosphorus, and unhealthy fats. Start with vegetables and fruits that are low in potassium, like cauliflower, bell peppers, blueberries, and grapes, making them the centerpiece of meals. These can be incorporated into dishes in a variety of ways, such as salads, steamed sides, or blended into smoothies, to add nutrients without overloading the kidneys.

Grains, particularly whole grains, should be selected carefully. Options like bulgur, buckwheat, and couscous are preferable as they offer fiber and are generally lower in phosphorus than other grains.

These can form the base of a meal, adding substance and satisfaction without compromising kidney health.

Protein intake needs careful management in CKD Stage 3. Lean proteins such as chicken, turkey, and fish are excellent choices. Plant-based proteins, including legumes and tofu, are also beneficial but should be chosen and portioned according to their potassium content. Cooking methods like grilling, broiling, or baking these proteins without adding salt or high-sodium sauces can help maintain the desired nutritional balance.

Dairy products and alternatives require attention as well. Opting for almond, rice, or soy-based products can reduce phosphorus and potassium intake while still providing the pleasure and nutritional benefits of dairy. When using these alternatives in cooking or baking, they can often be substituted directly for their dairy counterparts.

Sodium intake is a crucial consideration in every aspect of meal preparation for CKD Stage 3. Instead of salt, herbs, spices, and salt-free blends can flavor dishes effectively without adding sodium. This switch not only supports kidney health but also enhances the natural flavors of food, encouraging a healthier palate.

Fluid management is an aspect of meal planning that might not be immediately obvious but is essential for those with CKD. Fluid intake includes not just beverages but also the water content in soups, fruits, and vegetables. Monitoring and adjusting fluid intake based on individual needs and current kidney function can prevent complications such as swelling and high blood pressure.

Lastly, meal preparation at home offers the opportunity to control portion sizes, an important aspect of managing CKD. Serving appropriate portions ensures that the intake of critical nutrients is balanced, helping to avoid the risk of overconsumption which can strain the kidneys further.

Adopting these strategies for cooking and preparing meals at home can make a significant difference in managing CKD Stage 3. It allows individuals to enjoy a variety of foods while adhering to dietary restrictions, ultimately contributing to slower progression of kidney disease and improved overall health.

Eating Out with CKD Stage 3

Eating out with Chronic Kidney Disease (CKD) Stage 3 presents unique challenges, as it requires navigating menus to find options that align with kidney-friendly dietary restrictions. However, with careful planning and strategic choices, dining out can still be a pleasurable experience without compromising kidney health. The key lies in understanding the CKD Stage 3 food list, which emphasizes low sodium, low potassium, and low phosphorus foods, along with moderate protein intake.

When planning to eat out, researching restaurants in advance can make a significant difference. Many establishments offer their menus online, providing an opportunity to review options and identify suitable dishes before even stepping foot inside. It's helpful to look for restaurants that cook meals to order, as they are often more accommodating to requests for modifications that make dishes more kidney-friendly.

Upon arriving at the restaurant, don't hesitate to communicate with the server about specific dietary needs. Requesting the preparation of meals without added salt or MSG can significantly reduce sodium intake, which is crucial for managing blood pressure and fluid balance in CKD. Asking for sauces and dressings on the side allows for controlling the amount consumed, effectively managing intake of sodium, potassium, and phosphorus.

Selecting dishes that naturally fit within the CKD Stage 3 diet can simplify the dining out experience. Grilled or baked lean proteins such as chicken, fish, or turkey are excellent choices, as they provide essential nutrients without overloading the kidneys. Steamed vegetables rather than those cooked with butter or sauce, and side salads with a light drizzle of dressing, are kidney-friendly options that can help fill out the meal.

It's also important to be mindful of portion sizes, particularly with protein. Eating more protein than the body needs can increase the burden on the kidneys, so it's advisable to stick to appropriate serving sizes—typically about the size of a palm for meat and choosing smaller or appetizer portions when available.

Beverage choices also play a significant role in managing CKD Stage 3. Water, lemon water, and other clear drinks are preferable over sodas, and specialty beverages that may contain added sugars, sodium, and phosphorus. For those who enjoy alcohol, it's critical to consult with a healthcare provider about safe consumption, as alcohol can affect kidney function and interact with medications.

In situations where high-potassium foods like potatoes are part of a meal, requesting a substitute such as white rice or asking for the potato to be double-boiled can reduce potassium levels, making the dish safer for kidney health. Similarly, avoiding or limiting bread and rolls, which may contain added phosphorus, can help keep phosphorus levels in check.

Ultimately, eating out with CKD Stage 3 requires a balance between vigilance and enjoyment. By making informed choices based on a solid understanding of the CKD Stage 3 food list and maintaining open communication with restaurant staff, individuals can enjoy dining out while effectively managing their kidney health. Regular consultation with a healthcare provider or dietitian can also provide personalized advice and support for navigating the complexities of eating out with CKD.

Sample Meal Plans

Creating a meal plan when managing Chronic Kidney Disease (CKD) Stage 3 involves careful consideration of nutrient intake to support kidney health while ensuring the diet remains enjoyable and diverse. A balanced meal plan for CKD Stage 3 focuses on controlling intake of sodium, potassium, phosphorus, and the right amount of high-quality protein. It also emphasizes the importance of including a variety of kidney-friendly foods that provide essential vitamins and minerals. Below is a sample meal plan that incorporates these dietary guidelines, offering meals and snacks that are both nutritious and flavorful.

For breakfast, consider starting the day with a bowl of cooked apple and cinnamon oatmeal made with water or almond milk. Pair it with a side of fresh blueberries and a slice of whole-grain toast topped with avocado, which is a healthy source of fats and low in potassium compared to other fruits. This meal provides a good balance of carbohydrates for energy, while the avocado offers a creamy texture and healthy fats without overloading the kidneys.

Lunch could be a chicken salad made with grilled chicken breast, mixed greens, cucumbers, and shredded carrots, dressed in a homemade vinaigrette made from olive oil and lemon juice. Avoid high-potassium vegetables and opt for a variety of low-potassium vegetables to keep the salad flavorful and kidney-friendly. Serve the salad with a side of white rice or couscous for a satisfying meal that's light yet fulfilling.

For an afternoon snack, a small apple or a few slices of pear with a handful of unsalted almonds offers a quick, simple, and nutritious option. This snack provides fiber, healthy fats, and protein without excess sodium or phosphorus, making it perfect for managing CKD.

Dinner can be a serving of baked salmon seasoned with herbs and lemon juice, accompanied by roasted cauliflower and a quinoa salad. Salmon is a great source of omega-3 fatty acids and provides high-quality protein in a kidney-friendly quantity. Cauliflower is a low-potassium alternative to potatoes or other high-potassium vegetables, and quinoa is a versatile grain that's high in protein and fiber, making it an excellent choice for CKD Stage 3.

For dessert or an evening snack, a serving of rice pudding made with rice, almond milk, cinnamon, and a touch of honey can satisfy sweet cravings without adding excessive phosphorus or potassium to the diet. This dessert is comforting, easy to make, and can be adjusted for sweetness and flavor without compromising kidney health.

It's important for individuals managing CKD Stage 3 to drink fluids in moderation and to consult with a healthcare provider for personalized advice on fluid intake, as needs can vary based on individual health status and kidney function.

This sample meal plan is designed to provide balanced nutrition that supports kidney health in CKD Stage 3, incorporating a variety of foods to make meals enjoyable and to ensure dietary restrictions do not compromise taste and satisfaction. Regular consultations with a dietitian specialized in CKD can help tailor meal plans further to meet individual nutritional needs and preferences, ensuring the diet remains effective in managing kidney health and overall well-being.

Recipes for CKD Stage 3

Breakfast Recipes

breakfast recipes tailored for Chronic Kidney Disease (CKD) Stage 3 involves carefully selecting ingredients that support kidney health while still being delicious and satisfying. Below are detailed recipes, including ingredients, nutritional information, instructions, and serving sizes, specifically designed for those managing CKD Stage 3.

Recipe	Ingredients	Nutritional Information	Instructions	Serving Size
Apple Cinnamon Oatmeal	- 1 cup water or almond milk,- ½ cup rolled oats,- 1 medium apple, peeled and diced,- ½ teaspoon cinnamon,- 1 tablespoon honey or maple syrup	Calories: 250, Protein: 5 g, Sodium: 30 mg, Potassium: 200 mg, Phosphorus: 150 mg	1. In a small pot, bring water or almond milk to a boil.,2. Add oats and reduce heat to simmer, cooking for 5 minutes.,3. Stir in diced apple and cinnamon,	1 serving

Recipe	Ingredients (optional)	Nutritional Information	Instructions	Serving Size
			cooking for another 5 minutes or until the apples soften.,4. Sweeten with honey or maple syrup if desired.	
Avocado Toast	- 2 slices of whole-grain bread,- 1 ripe avocado,- Lemon juice (to taste),- Pinch of salt (optional)	Calories: 300, Protein: 9 g, Sodium: 200 mg, Potassium: 500 mg, Phosphorus: 100 mg	1. Toast the bread slices to your preference.,2. In a bowl, mash the avocado and mix in a little lemon juice and salt if desired.,3. Spread the mashed	2 slices

Recipe	Ingredients	Nutritional Information	Instructions	Serving Size
			avocado evenly on the toasted bread slices.	
Berry Smoothie	- ½ cup blueberries,- ½ cup strawberries,- 1 cup almond milk,- ½ cup ice,- 1 tablespoon honey (optional)	Calories: 150, Protein: 2 g, Sodium: 80 mg, Potassium: 150 mg, Phosphorus: 50 mg	1. In a blender, combine blueberries, strawberries, almond milk, and ice.,2. Blend until smooth.,3. Add honey to sweeten if desired and blend again until mixed well.	1 serving

Recipe	Ingredients	Nutritional Information	Instructions	Serving Size
Egg White Scramble	- 4 egg whites,- ½ cup chopped spinach,- ½ cup diced bell peppers,- 1 tablespoon olive oil,- Salt and pepper to taste	Calories: 150, Protein: 15 g, Sodium: 170 mg, Potassium: 220 mg, Phosphorus: 70 mg	1. Heat olive oil in a non-stick skillet over medium heat.,2. Add bell peppers and sauté until soft, about 3-4 minutes.,3. Add spinach and cook until wilted.,4. Pour in egg whites, stirring gently until they are fully cooked. Season with salt and pepper.	1 serving

These recipes are designed to be kidney-friendly for individuals with CKD Stage 3, focusing on limiting sodium, potassium, and phosphorus intake while providing adequate protein and calories for a nutritious start to the day. Adjustments can be made based on individual dietary needs and preferences, and it's always recommended to consult with a healthcare provider or dietitian when making significant changes to your diet, especially when managing a health condition like CKD.

Lunch Recipes

Each recipe is tailored to ensure it meets dietary guidelines for sodium, potassium, and phosphorus content, while providing delicious and nutritious options. The table includes ingredients, nutritional information, instructions, and serving sizes for each recipe.

Recipe	Ingredients	Nutritional Information (per serving)	Instructions	Serving Size
Grilled Chicken and Veggie Wrap	- 2 whole-grain tortillas,- 6 oz grilled chicken breast, sliced,- 1 cup shredded lettuce,- 1/4 cup shredded carrots,- 1/4	Calories: 350, Protein: 28 g, Sodium: 200 mg, Potassium: 400 mg, Phosphorus: 250 mg	1. Lay out the tortillas on a flat surface.,2. Evenly distribute chicken, lettuce, carrots, and cucumbers on each tortilla.,3.	2 servings

Recipe	Ingredients	Nutritional Information (per serving)	Instructions	Serving Size
	cup diced cucumbers,- 2 tbsp low-sodium dressing		Drizzle with low-sodium dressing.,4. Roll up the tortillas tightly to enclose the filling.,5. Serve immediately or wrap in foil to keep fresh.	
Quinoa Salad with Lemon Herb Dressing	- 1 cup cooked quinoa,- 1/2 cup diced bell peppers,- 1/4 cup	Calories: 220, Protein: 6 g, Sodium: 30 mg, Potassium: 320 mg,	1. In a large bowl, combine cooked quinoa, bell peppers, red onion, and	4 servings

Recipe	Ingredients	Nutritional Information (per serving)	Instructions	Serving Size
	chopped red onion,- 1/4 cup chopped parsley,- 2 tbsp olive oil,- Juice of 1 lemon,- 1 tsp dried oregano,- Salt and pepper to taste	Phosphorus: 150 mg	parsley.,2. In a small bowl, whisk together olive oil, lemon juice, oregano, salt, and pepper.,3. Pour the dressing over the quinoa mixture and toss to combine.,4. Chill in the refrigerator for at least 30 minutes	

Recipe	Ingredients	Nutritional Information (per serving)	Instructions	Serving Size
			before serving to allow flavors to meld.	
Tuna Salad Stuffed Avocado	- 2 medium avocados, halved and pitted,- 4 oz canned low-sodium tuna, drained,- 1/4 cup diced celery,- 1/4 cup diced apple,- 2 tbsp mayonnaise,- 1 tsp lemon juice,- Salt and pepper	Calories: 290, Protein: 14 g, Sodium: 140 mg, Potassium: 500 mg, Phosphorus: 200 mg	1. In a bowl, mix together tuna, celery, apple, mayonnaise, lemon juice, salt, and pepper.,2. Scoop out some of the avocado flesh to create more space, leaving a thin layer	4 servings

Recipe	Ingredients	Nutritional Information (per serving)	Instructions	Serving Size
	to taste		inside the skin.,3. Fill each avocado half with the tuna mixture.,4. Serve immediately or chill for a short period before serving.	
Vegetable Stir-Fry with Brown Rice	- 1 cup cooked brown rice,- 2 cups mixed vegetables (e.g., broccoli,	Calories: 320, Protein: 8 g, Sodium: 150 mg, Potassium: 450 mg, Phosphorus:	1. Heat olive oil in a large skillet over medium heat.,2. Add garlic and ginger, sautéing for	2 servings

Recipe	Ingredients	Nutritional Information (per serving)	Instructions	Serving Size
	carrots, bell peppers), thinly sliced,- 2 tbsp low-sodium soy sauce,- 1 tbsp olive oil,- 1 tsp garlic, minced,- 1 tsp ginger, minced,- 1 tbsp sesame seeds (optional)	220 mg	1 minute until fragrant.,3. Add the mixed vegetables and stir-fry for 5-7 minutes until tender-crisp.,4. Stir in the low-sodium soy sauce and cook for another minute.,5. Serve the vegetable stir-fry over	

Recipe	Ingredients	Nutritional Information (per serving)	Instructions	Serving Size
			cooked brown rice., 6. Sprinkle with sesame seeds if desired.	

These lunch recipes are designed to be both nutritious and satisfying, with careful attention to the dietary restrictions associated with CKD Stage 3. Each recipe provides a balanced meal option, focusing on limiting ingredients that are high in sodium, potassium, and phosphorus, which are important considerations for individuals with kidney disease. Always consult with a healthcare provider or dietitian to ensure these meals fit within your specific dietary needs.

Dinner Recipes

These recipes provide a variety of flavors and nutrients without overloading the kidneys with high levels of sodium, potassium, phosphorus, or excessive protein.

Recipe Name	Ingredients	Nutritional Information (per serving)	Instructions	Serving Size
Herb-Baked Fish	- 4 oz tilapia fillets,- 2 tbsp olive oil,- 1 tsp dried basil,- 1 tsp dried thyme,- ½ tsp garlic powder,- Lemon wedges for garnish	Calories: 220, Protein: 23 g, Sodium: 70 mg, Potassium: 370 mg, Phosphorus: 250 mg	1. Preheat oven to 375°F.,2. Mix olive oil, basil, thyme, and garlic powder in a bowl.,3. Brush the mixture over the tilapia fillets.,4. Place fillets in a baking dish and bake for 12-15 minutes, until	1 serving

Recipe Name	Ingredients	Nutritional Information (per serving)	Instructions	Serving Size
			fish flakes easily with a fork.,5. Serve with lemon wedges.	
Quinoa Stuffed Bell Peppers	- 2 large bell peppers, halved and seeded,- 1 cup cooked quinoa,- 1 cup diced tomatoes, no added salt,- ¼ cup chopped onions,- ¼ cup shredded	Calories: 190, Protein: 8 g, Sodium: 85 mg, Potassium: 410 mg, Phosphorus: 150 mg	1. Preheat oven to 350°F.,2. In a skillet, heat olive oil and sauté onions until translucent.,3. Add tomatoes, cumin, and paprika. Cook for 5 minutes.,4. Stir	2 servings

105 | CKD STAGE 3 FOOD LIST

Recipe Name	Ingredients	Nutritional Information (per serving)	Instructions	Serving Size
	mozzarella cheese,- 1 tbsp olive oil,- 1 tsp cumin,- 1 tsp paprika		in cooked quinoa.,5. Stuff the bell peppers with the quinoa mixture and top with cheese.,6. Bake for 25-30 minutes.	
Chicken and Vegetable Stir-Fry	- 4 oz chicken breast, thinly sliced,- 1 cup broccoli florets,- ½ cup sliced carrots,- ½ cup snow peas,- 2 tbsp low-sodium soy sauce,- 1	Calories: 240, Protein: 26 g, Sodium: 330 mg, Potassium: 495 mg, Phosphorus: 220 mg	1. Heat olive oil in a large pan over medium heat.,2. Add garlic and ginger, sauté for 1 minute.,3. Add chicken and cook until no longer pink.,4. Add	1 serving

Recipe Name	Ingredients	Nutritional Information (per serving)	Instructions	Serving Size
	tbsp olive oil,- 1 garlic clove, minced,- 1 tsp ginger, grated		broccoli, carrots, and snow peas. Cook for 5-7 minutes, until vegetables are tender-crisp.,5. Stir in soy sauce and cook for another 2 minutes.	
Lemon Garlic Pasta with Zucchini	- 2 cups cooked spaghetti, whole wheat,- 1 cup zucchini, sliced,- 2 tbsp olive oil,- 2 garlic cloves,	Calories: 320, Protein: 11 g, Sodium: 120 mg, Potassium: 275 mg, Phosphorus: 150 mg	1. In a skillet, heat olive oil over medium heat.,2. Add garlic and zucchini. Sauté until zucchini is tender.,3. Add cooked	2 servings

Recipe Name	Ingredients	Nutritional Information (per serving)	Instructions	Serving Size
	minced,- Juice of 1 lemon,- 2 tbsp grated Parmesan cheese,- 1 tbsp fresh parsley, chopped		spaghetti, lemon juice, and toss well.,4. Garnish with Parmesan cheese and fresh parsley before serving.	

These recipes are designed to be adaptable for those managing CKD Stage 3, with careful consideration of ingredient choices to ensure they are kidney-friendly while still delicious and satisfying. Remember, it's important to consult with a healthcare provider or dietitian when making dietary changes, especially for those with CKD, to tailor meal plans and recipes to individual health needs and dietary restrictions.

Snack and Dessert Recipes

Creating snack and dessert recipes suitable for individuals with Chronic Kidney Disease (CKD) Stage 3 involves careful selection of ingredients to manage intake of potassium, phosphorus, sodium, and protein. Here are two recipes that fit within the dietary guidelines for CKD Stage 3, providing enjoyable options that are kidney-friendly.

Recipe	Ingredients	Nutritional Information (per serving)	Instructions	Serving Size
Almond and Berry Salad	- 1 cup mixed berries (blueberries, strawberries, raspberries) , - ¼ cup slivered almonds , - 1 tablespoon honey , - 1	Calories: 150 , Sodium: 5 mg , Potassium: 200 mg , Phosphorus: 100 mg , Protein: 4 g	1. In a mixing bowl, combine the mixed berries. , 2. In a small bowl, whisk together honey and lemon juice until well blended. , 3.	2 servings

109 | CKD STAGE 3 FOOD LIST

Recipe	Ingredients	Nutritional Information (per serving)	Instructions	Serving Size
	teaspoon fresh lemon juice		Drizzle the honey and lemon mixture over the berries and gently toss to coat. , 4. Sprinkle slivered almonds on top before serving.	
Rice Pudding with Cinnamon	- ½ cup uncooked white rice , - 2 cups almond milk , - ¼ teaspoon salt , - ¼	Calories: 220 , Sodium: 80 mg , Potassium: 90 mg , Phosphorus: 60 mg , Protein: 3 g	1. In a saucepan, combine rice, almond milk, and salt. Bring to a boil over medium	4 servings

Recipe	Ingredients	Nutritional Information (per serving)	Instructions	Serving Size
	cup sugar, - ½ teaspoon vanilla extract, - ½ teaspoon cinnamon		heat. , 2. Reduce heat to low and simmer, covered, until rice is tender and most of the liquid is absorbed, about 20-25 minutes. , 3. Stir in sugar, vanilla extract, and cinnamon. Cook for another 5 minutes. , 4. Remove	

Recipe	Ingredients	Nutritional Information (per serving)	Instructions	Serving Size
			from heat and let it cool slightly. It will thicken as it cools. , 5. Serve warm or chilled.	

These recipes provide kidney-friendly snack and dessert options for individuals managing CKD Stage 3. The almond and berry salad offers a refreshing and nutritious snack with a good balance of sweetness, acidity, and crunch, while keeping the potassium and phosphorus content in check. The rice pudding is a comforting and versatile dessert that can be adjusted in sweetness according to preference, providing a low-potassium and low-phosphorus treat. Both recipes emphasize the importance of portion control and balance in the diet of individuals with CKD Stage.

Managing CKD Stage 3 with Diet

Adjusting to Dietary Changes

Adjusting to dietary changes is a crucial aspect of managing Chronic Kidney Disease (CKD) Stage 3, as it involves a shift in eating habits to support kidney health and slow the progression of the disease. This process can be challenging but also empowering, as individuals learn to make informed choices about their nutrition. The goal is to limit intake of certain nutrients that are harder for damaged kidneys to process, such as sodium, potassium, phosphorus, and certain amounts of protein, while ensuring a balanced intake of calories, vitamins, and minerals to maintain overall health.

Initially, understanding which foods to choose and which to avoid can seem daunting. A CKD Stage 3 food list is an invaluable tool, providing a clear guide to kidney-friendly foods. This list typically highlights fruits and vegetables with lower potassium levels, lean proteins, grains, and options for dairy or dairy alternatives with low phosphorus content. Learning to read food labels for sodium, potassium, and phosphorus content becomes a necessary skill, enabling individuals to make smarter choices when shopping and eating out.

Incorporating these dietary changes often requires a shift in cooking and eating habits. Cooking at home becomes more of a necessity, as it allows for better control over ingredients and portion sizes. Experimenting with herbs and spices can offer new flavors and enjoyment in meals, replacing the reliance on salt for seasoning. Planning meals ahead and preparing kidney-friendly dishes can make adhering to dietary guidelines more manageable and less time-consuming.

One of the biggest adjustments may come from modifying protein intake. High-quality protein sources like fish, egg whites, and chicken are recommended in controlled amounts. Balancing protein intake involves understanding how much protein is needed to maintain health while not overburdening the kidneys.

Dealing with restrictions on potassium and phosphorus intake means rethinking fruit and vegetable choices, as well as nuts, seeds, and dairy products. Emphasizing lower-potassium fruits and vegetables and seeking alternatives to high-phosphorus foods like certain dairy products can help maintain a varied and enjoyable diet.

Social situations and dining out present their own challenges, as food choices are more limited. It can be helpful to preview restaurant menus online to identify kidney-friendly options or to suggest dining locations that offer suitable choices. Being open with friends and family about dietary needs can garner support and understanding, making social meals more enjoyable.

The emotional and psychological aspects of dietary changes should not be underestimated. It's normal to experience frustration, resistance, or sadness as familiar foods may need to be limited or avoided. However, many find that their tastes adapt over time, and discovering new foods and recipes can be a rewarding experience.

Support from dietitians, healthcare providers, and kidney disease support groups can be incredibly beneficial. These resources can offer personalized advice, practical tips, and emotional support to navigate dietary changes. Learning from others who are facing similar challenges can provide encouragement and a sense of community.

Ultimately, adjusting to dietary changes in CKD Stage 3 is a gradual process that involves education, experimentation, and adaptation. It's about making informed choices that support kidney health without sacrificing the pleasure of eating. With the right resources and support, individuals can successfully manage their diet, contributing to their overall well-being and quality of life while living with CKD.

Monitoring Your Health and Kidney Function

Monitoring health and kidney function is a critical component of managing Chronic Kidney Disease (CKD) Stage 3, especially when dietary adjustments are a primary strategy for slowing disease progression. As CKD Stage 3 marks a moderate decline in kidney function, regular check-ups with healthcare providers, including nephrologists and dietitians, become essential for tracking the effectiveness of dietary management and making necessary adjustments.

One of the key measures of kidney function is the glomerular filtration rate (GFR), which estimates the rate at which kidneys are filtering blood. A decline in GFR indicates worsening kidney function, prompting a review and possible modification of dietary plans. Blood pressure monitoring is also vital since hypertension can both cause and result from kidney damage. Maintaining blood pressure within recommended levels through diet, exercise, and medication can help protect kidney function.

Blood tests play a significant role in monitoring CKD. These tests measure levels of creatinine, urea, and other waste products that kidneys filter out. Elevated levels can indicate a reduction in kidney function. Electrolyte balance, particularly potassium and phosphorus levels, is closely watched because imbalances can lead to serious health issues. Potassium is critical for heart function, and too much can lead to irregular heartbeats or heart attack, while excess phosphorus can lead to bone and cardiovascular problems.

Dietitians often recommend keeping a food diary as part of dietary management for CKD Stage 3. This tool can help individuals track their intake of nutrients that need to be limited, such as sodium, potassium, and phosphorus, and ensure they are getting adequate but not excessive protein. A food diary can also be useful for identifying foods or meals that may contribute to any imbalances or health issues, allowing for timely adjustments to the diet.

In addition to regular healthcare visits and blood tests, individuals with CKD Stage 3 should monitor their body for signs of fluid retention, such as swelling in the legs, ankles, or around the eyes, which can indicate the kidneys are struggling to remove excess fluid from the body. Monitoring weight can help identify sudden increases due to fluid retention.

Dietary management also includes ensuring adequate calorie intake to maintain a healthy weight, as malnutrition can be a concern in later stages of CKD. Adequate intake of vitamins and minerals, within kidney-friendly limits, supports overall health. Supplements may be necessary, but only under the guidance of healthcare providers, as some vitamins and minerals can accumulate to dangerous levels in CKD.

Lastly, self-monitoring for symptoms of CKD progression, such as fatigue, changes in urination patterns, and difficulty concentrating, is important. Promptly reporting these changes to healthcare providers can help in adjusting treatment plans, including dietary management, to better support kidney function and overall health.

In managing CKD Stage 3 with diet, the goal is to balance nutrient intake to support kidney health and slow disease progression while maintaining overall well-being. Regular monitoring of health and kidney function, in partnership with healthcare providers, is essential to navigate this balance effectively.

When to Consult Your Healthcare Provider

Managing Chronic Kidney Disease (CKD) Stage 3 through diet is a delicate balance that requires careful monitoring and adjustments over time. While a kidney-friendly food list and dietary guidelines serve as valuable tools in slowing the progression of CKD, it's essential to recognize situations that warrant professional medical advice. Consulting with a healthcare provider is crucial not only for dietary management but also for overseeing the overall treatment plan for CKD.

Signs and symptoms indicating the need for medical consultation can vary but typically include an increase in fatigue or a decrease in energy levels, which could suggest anemia or worsening kidney function. Changes in urinary habits, such as an increase or decrease in frequency, the presence of blood, or foamy urine, should prompt immediate discussion with a healthcare provider, as these can be signs of progressing kidney damage.

Swelling or edema, especially in the legs, ankles, or around the eyes, is another key indicator that kidney function may be declining. This swelling is due to the kidneys' decreased ability to manage fluid and salt balances. High blood pressure is a common complication of

CKD and requires careful management; sudden changes in blood pressure readings, whether higher or lower, necessitate a consultation with a healthcare provider to adjust medication or dietary salt intake accordingly.

For individuals managing CKD Stage 3, monitoring for signs of electrolyte imbalances, such as hyperkalemia (high potassium levels) or hyperphosphatemia (high phosphorus levels), is crucial. Symptoms can include muscle cramps, weakness, and in severe cases, irregular heart rhythms. Given the dietary restrictions on potassium and phosphorus in CKD, any unusual symptoms should be discussed with a healthcare provider to determine if dietary adjustments or medication are needed.

Unexpected weight loss or gain can also indicate that the dietary management of CKD needs reevaluation. Weight loss might suggest inadequate calorie or protein intake, while weight gain could indicate fluid retention, both of which require medical advice to ensure the diet meets nutritional needs without exacerbating kidney damage.

Moreover, if there's difficulty adhering to the dietary restrictions or confusion about the kidney-friendly food list, seeking guidance from a dietitian specialized in renal diets is advisable. They can provide personalized advice and adjustments to the diet plan, ensuring it is balanced, nutritionally adequate, and sustainable in the long term.

Lastly, regular follow-ups with a healthcare provider are essential for monitoring kidney function and the effectiveness of the dietary management plan. These appointments are opportunities to discuss any concerns, review blood test results, and make necessary adjustments to the treatment plan based on the progression of CKD.

Managing CKD Stage 3 with diet is a proactive approach that involves continuous monitoring of one's health and symptoms. Recognizing when to seek medical advice is critical in effectively managing the condition and preventing its progression. Regular consultations with healthcare providers and dietitians ensure that dietary management remains tailored to the individual's changing needs, supporting overall health and kidney function.

Supplements and Medications

Understanding the Role of Supplements

When managing Chronic Kidney Disease (CKD) Stage 3, the role of dietary supplements becomes a significant consideration due to the body's changing needs and the kidneys' decreased ability to filter and maintain the balance of nutrients. Supplements can either be beneficial or potentially harmful, depending on their type, dosage, and the individual's specific health conditions. It is crucial for patients with CKD Stage 3 to have a clear understanding of which supplements may be necessary to support their health, as well as those that could exacerbate their condition.

In CKD Stage 3, the kidneys are moderately impaired. They may not adequately excrete certain minerals, leading to imbalances. For example, phosphorus levels can become too high, as the kidneys lose their ability to eliminate excess phosphorus from the blood. This imbalance can pull calcium out of the bones, making them weak. To manage this, healthcare providers may recommend phosphorus binders, a type of supplement that helps the body eliminate excess phosphorus. However, these are technically more medication than supplement and must be prescribed.

Vitamin D levels also need careful management in CKD Stage 3. The kidneys play a vital role in converting vitamin D to its active form, which is crucial for calcium absorption and bone health. As kidney function declines, so does the conversion of vitamin D, potentially leading to bone disease and other complications. Supplementing with vitamin D may be advised, but again, under medical supervision to avoid toxicity, as vitamin D levels can accumulate to dangerous levels in the body.

Anemia is another concern in CKD, as the diseased kidneys often produce less erythropoietin, a hormone needed for making red blood cells. This condition might necessitate iron supplements or vitamin B12 and folic acid, which are vital for red blood cell production. Yet, iron supplements should be carefully monitored as they can contribute to elevated levels of phosphorus and potassium.

While some supplements are necessary to manage the complications of CKD Stage 3, others can be harmful. For example, over-the-counter supplements containing potassium, magnesium, and herbal supplements that claim to boost kidney health can be dangerous for CKD patients. High levels of potassium can cause heart problems, while excessive magnesium can lead to its accumulation in the body due to the kidneys' reduced ability to excrete it.

The necessity of omega-3 fatty acid supplements in CKD Stage 3 diet management is debated. Omega-3s, found in fish oil, have anti-inflammatory properties and may help manage blood pressure and lipid levels. However, consuming omega-3s through diet by eating kidney-friendly fish options is generally preferred over supplementation to avoid the risk of consuming too much and affecting blood clotting.

It is vital for individuals with CKD Stage 3 to work closely with their healthcare team, including nephrologists and dietitians, before starting any new supplement. The management of CKD Stage 3 involves a delicate balance of nutrients, and what is beneficial in one stage of kidney disease might be harmful in another. A healthcare provider can help navigate these complexities by recommending supplements based on blood work, nutritional needs, and overall health status, ensuring that supplementation supports kidney health without causing additional harm.

Common Medications and Their Dietary Implications

Managing Chronic Kidney Disease (CKD) Stage 3 often requires the use of medications to control symptoms and slow the progression of the disease. Alongside dietary management, understanding the interplay between medications and nutrition is crucial for maintaining overall health and kidney function. Many common medications prescribed for CKD and its associated conditions can have significant dietary implications, necessitating adjustments to food choices and nutrient intake.

Phosphate binders are frequently prescribed to manage phosphorus levels in the blood, a common issue in CKD patients. These medications bind to phosphorus in the gastrointestinal tract, preventing its absorption. Patients on phosphate binders may need to monitor their intake of phosphorus-rich foods like dairy products, nuts, and seeds, even though these foods are part of a balanced diet, to avoid counteracting the medication's effects.

Blood pressure medications, including ACE inhibitors and ARBs, are often used to manage hypertension in CKD patients. While these medications can slow the progression of kidney disease, they may increase potassium levels in the blood. Therefore, individuals on these medications might need to limit high-potassium foods, such as bananas, oranges, potatoes, and tomatoes, to prevent hyperkalemia, a condition where potassium levels in the blood are too high.

Diuretics, or water pills, help remove excess fluid from the body, a common issue in CKD. Depending on the type of diuretic, they can either increase or decrease the excretion of potassium. Those on potassium-sparing diuretics should be cautious with high-potassium foods, while those on loop or thiazide diuretics may need to ensure adequate potassium intake from low-potassium sources like apples, carrots, and green beans.

Erythropoiesis-stimulating agents (ESAs) are used to treat anemia by stimulating the bone marrow to produce more red blood cells. For patients on ESAs, adequate iron intake is essential to support the production of red blood cells. However, iron supplements should be taken under medical supervision to avoid iron overload, which can be harmful to the kidneys. Iron-rich foods that are also low in potassium and phosphorus, such as egg whites and lean meats, can be beneficial.

Vitamin D supplements may be necessary for CKD Stage 3 patients to manage bone health and prevent renal osteodystrophy, a bone disorder resulting from impaired kidney function. While vitamin D is vital, it's important to monitor calcium intake through the diet, as excessive calcium can lead to vascular calcification and other complications in CKD patients.

Finally, nonsteroidal anti-inflammatory drugs (NSAIDs) should be used with caution in CKD patients, as they can further impair kidney function. While not directly related to diet, the use of NSAIDs highlights the importance of overall health management in CKD, including dietary considerations.

For CKD Stage 3 patients, managing diet and medication together is essential for optimal health outcomes. This often requires the guidance of a healthcare team, including a nephrologist and a dietitian, to tailor dietary advice and medication management to individual needs, ensuring both safety and nutritional adequacy.

Lifestyle Considerations

Exercise and Physical Activity

Exercise and physical activity are crucial components of managing Chronic Kidney Disease (CKD) Stage 3, complementing dietary considerations to enhance overall health and slow the progression of the disease. Regular physical activity helps improve cardiovascular health, control blood pressure, maintain a healthy weight, and reduce stress, all of which are important for individuals with CKD.

Incorporating exercise into the lifestyle of someone with CKD Stage 3 requires careful consideration of the type, intensity, and duration of physical activities to ensure they are safe and beneficial. Walking, cycling, swimming, and light resistance training are excellent choices that can be adjusted to fit individual fitness levels and health conditions. These activities are low impact, reducing the risk of injury, and can be easily integrated into daily routines.

Walking is a highly accessible form of exercise that requires no special equipment and can be performed almost anywhere. Starting with short walks and gradually increasing the distance and pace can help build endurance and cardiovascular health without overstraining the body. Cycling, either stationary or on a bike, offers cardiovascular benefits and strengthens the lower body with minimal stress on the joints. Swimming provides a full-body workout, improving muscle strength and flexibility while the buoyancy of the water reduces the risk of injury. Light resistance training, using body weight or light weights, can help maintain muscle mass, which is often a concern for individuals with CKD due to dietary protein restrictions.

It's important for individuals with CKD Stage 3 to begin any new exercise regimen under the guidance of healthcare professionals. They can provide personalized advice based on current health status, kidney function, and any other existing health issues. Monitoring how the body responds to exercise is crucial, and activities should be adjusted based on any changes in health or energy levels.

Nutrition plays a key role in supporting physical activity for individuals with CKD Stage 3. The CKD Stage 3 food list, emphasizing controlled intake of potassium, phosphorus, sodium, and protein, also needs to support the increased energy demands of regular exercise. Adequate intake of calories and nutrients is essential to fuel physical activity and support recovery and muscle repair afterward. Including a variety of kidney-friendly carbohydrates for energy, such as rice, pasta, and bread, along with lean proteins for muscle repair, and a wide range of fruits and vegetables for vitamins and minerals, ensures a well-rounded diet.

Hydration is another critical aspect, especially for individuals engaging in regular exercise. Fluid needs can vary greatly among individuals with CKD, and it's important to balance staying hydrated with avoiding fluid overload, which can strain the kidneys. Monitoring fluid intake and adjusting based on exercise intensity and duration, as well as individual fluid restrictions, is necessary.

Exercise and physical activity are integral to managing CKD Stage 3, offering numerous benefits that complement dietary management. A carefully planned approach, considering the type and intensity of exercise and nutritional support, can enhance quality of life and potentially slow the progression of CKD. Regular consultation with healthcare providers ensures that exercise and dietary plans are tailored to individual needs, making them safe, effective, and sustainable.

Managing Stress and Mental Health

Managing stress and mental health is crucial for individuals with Chronic Kidney Disease (CKD) Stage 3, as the diagnosis and lifestyle changes required can be significant sources of emotional distress. Stress can exacerbate CKD symptoms and complications, making it essential to adopt strategies that promote mental well-being alongside physical health management, including adherence to a CKD Stage 3 food list.

Stress management techniques are varied and can be personalized to fit one's lifestyle and preferences. Mindfulness meditation, for example, has been shown to reduce stress by encouraging a state of active, open attention to the present. Practicing mindfulness can help individuals with CKD become more aware of their bodies, thoughts, and feelings in the moment, potentially reducing anxiety and improving their ability to cope with the disease.

Regular physical activity, tailored to the individual's abilities and recommended by a healthcare provider, can also play a significant role in managing stress. Exercise releases endorphins, which are natural mood lifters, and can improve sleep quality, which in turn, can reduce stress levels. Activities such as walking, swimming, or yoga can be particularly beneficial for those with CKD, offering gentle but effective ways to stay active.

Support groups offer another avenue for stress relief, providing a platform for sharing experiences and coping strategies with others facing similar challenges. These groups can be found through hospitals, kidney foundations, or online communities. Sharing experiences and tips, including those related to following a CKD Stage 3 food list, can provide emotional support and practical advice, reducing feelings of isolation and anxiety.

Dietary management is also linked to mental health; a balanced diet can impact mood and energy levels. For individuals with CKD Stage 3, adhering to a kidney-friendly food list not only supports physical health but can also contribute to a sense of control and empowerment over one's health, potentially reducing stress. Incorporating a variety of nutritious foods that align with dietary restrictions can help ensure the diet remains enjoyable, which is important for overall well-being.

Professional counseling or therapy can be beneficial for individuals dealing with chronic illnesses like CKD. Cognitive-behavioral therapy (CBT), in particular, can help modify negative thought patterns and develop coping strategies for dealing with stress and the emotional aspects of living with a chronic condition.

It's important for individuals with CKD and their families to recognize the signs of depression and anxiety, which can include persistent sadness, loss of interest in activities, changes in sleep or appetite, and feelings of hopelessness. Early intervention is key to managing these conditions effectively, so seeking help from a mental health professional should be encouraged if these symptoms arise.

Managing stress and mental health for individuals with CKD Stage 3 involves a holistic approach that incorporates mindfulness, physical activity, support networks, dietary management, and professional counseling when necessary. These strategies not only support mental well-being but can also have a positive impact on physical health, creating a comprehensive approach to managing CKD.

Conclusion

Concluding a guide on the dietary management for individuals with Chronic Kidney Disease (CKD) at Stage 3, it's crucial to emphasize the importance of a balanced, kidney-friendly diet in slowing disease progression and managing symptoms. At this stage of CKD, the kidneys are moderately impaired, making it essential to adjust dietary intake to support kidney health and prevent further damage.

The cornerstone of a Stage 3 CKD diet is moderation and balance. It involves limiting certain nutrients that can exacerbate kidney damage while ensuring adequate intake of others to maintain overall health. Key dietary adjustments include:

1. **Protein Moderation**: While protein is a vital nutrient, excessive consumption can strain the kidneys. It's advisable to consume moderate amounts of high-quality protein, focusing on plant-based sources and lean meats to minimize kidney stress.

2. **Phosphorus and Calcium Balance**: High phosphorus levels can lead to bone health issues. Foods rich in phosphorus, such as dairy products, nuts, and seeds, should be consumed in moderation. Calcium intake should be balanced to support bone health, with guidance from healthcare professionals to adjust for individual needs.

3. **Potassium Regulation**: Depending on the stage of CKD and the individual's blood test results, potassium intake may need to be adjusted. High-potassium foods may need to be limited to avoid dangerous changes in blood potassium levels, affecting heart health.

4. **Sodium and Fluid Control**: Reducing sodium intake can help manage blood pressure and swelling, common issues in CKD. Limiting foods high in salt and monitoring fluid intake can prevent fluid overload, which can stress the heart and kidneys.

5. **Healthy Fats**: Incorporating healthy fats, such as those from fish, olive oil, and avocados, can support heart health without overburdening the kidneys.

6. **Fiber**: A diet high in fiber from fruits, vegetables, and whole grains can help manage CKD symptoms and improve overall digestive health.

7. **Individualized Nutrient Adjustments**: It's important to work with a healthcare team, including a dietitian, to make personalized dietary adjustments based on the progression of CKD, laboratory results, and individual health goals.

In conclusion, managing diet in Stage 3 CKD involves careful consideration of nutrient intake to support kidney function, prevent further damage, and maintain overall health. By adhering to a kidney-friendly diet, individuals can play a crucial role in managing their CKD, improving their quality of life, and potentially slowing the progression of the disease. Regular consultations with healthcare providers are essential to tailor dietary recommendations to the individual's needs, monitor health status, and adjust dietary plans as necessary.

www.ingramcontent.com/pod-product-compliance
Lightning Source LLC
Chambersburg PA
CBHW071057240526
45471CB00016B/1986